Adventures in Careland

ISBN: 1-4538-9992-8
ISBN-13: 9781453899922

Adventures in Careland

Façades and Back Rooms
of Institutionalized Aging
Gilah Silber M.D.

2011

Dedication

The Silber Principle—A Series of Chaotic Events that Led to the Perfect Relationship

As your alter ego, I mirror your body and spirit. Thus I multitask and compose the dedication of my second book and a tribute to you, my *beshart*, on your fiftieth birthday. The exercise brings life to a standstill as I recall our trials and tribulations. You have supported me through everything, including my latest aspirations as an author. With our time together at a premium, the book project turned leisure moments from rare to nonexistent. Your only complaint was that you wanted "more of me." I write now to respond a little to that request. Yet, as we often tell each other, "no good deed goes unpunished." As I write, I find myself going against my principles of style in wanting to compose no ordinary dedication but something sentimental—a love letter—not just a brief nod in print.

The most important things in life are unforeseen and unforeseeable. For us, it was our chance meeting in a small office at an undisclosed university. The details of how we met still amaze me. If we could develop a convincing way to tell the truth, our story could be a best seller. At the very least, it might make an atheist question his or her philosophy. That first meeting sealed our fate. Life, as we now know it, began; the formative period occurred in the first few months thereafter.

I can highlight our twenty-four years together in a paragraph. We met and married within a year. You earned a doctorate and began your career as a computer scientist (a career you maintain to this day). We moved and bought a home. I went to medical school. We birthed a daughter, and moved to a new home (where we still reside). I started a residency. We birthed a son. I started a fellowship and a medical practice. We birthed another daughter. We divorced. Yes, the pain and discord were unforeseen. Yet it must've been then that you morphed into the Abe Silber with whom I'm proud to share my life. Fourteen months later, we remarried—in a Las Vegas quickie—and found happiness the second time around.

Now after almost a quarter-century together, how do I attempt to describe you? You're the same, with only a few of the details changed—for the better. You're a genius, with such intelligence that I've never remotely seen surpassed. You make me laugh. You are as great a father as you are a husband. You learn from your mistakes and take honesty and ethics to new levels. You're a great athlete and have a body that a twenty-one-year-old man would envy. You never had to shed your "old country" ways, because to me you've never been foreign. Our psyches are ninety-five percent alike. The remaining five percent does not breed conflict so much as stimulation. How's that for match.com?

Thanks for more than a few big things that I never had before we met: security and confidence, love, a family, a home, and trust in life. Thanks for the many somewhat smaller things: fixing the computer, driving us on many long, family trips, and giving freely of your time to tend to the children and me. Thanks for the millions of tiny things: doing laundry and washing dishes, telling me what wine I like, giving me the right coffee cup, moving furniture, buying the perfect jewelry, getting me a double-sided printer and an electric stapler, and loving my cooking as well as my housekeeping and decorating. Last but not least—organizing the trash!

We've been through a whirlwind. We can officially say that we're not in Kansas anymore. In light of our multiple hardships, which are best stored in the deeper crevices of our brains—not to be forgotten but not to be dwelled on—I'll mention another favorite phrase: "That which does not kill us makes us stronger."

You're the greatest.

L'chaim!

May we live to be one hundred and twenty.

With love and devotion forever,

It's been a hell of a ride.

GS

August 19, 2008

Contents

Acknowledgment

With many thanks and great appreciation
to my editor, Marie France

Preface

On the Frontlines of Aging

As a practicing geriatric physician, I am disheartened to see good intentions do more harm than good as we seek to improve the way that we care for our aged and infirm. Vocal, concerned, and proactive individuals—many of them baby boomers—express dissatisfaction with the long-term care facilities in which they place their loved ones. They want institutions that are less institutional in nature. They also want ones that operate as close to zero risk as humanly possible.

Asked to become homier, nursing homes have responded by adopting a number of new practices in recent years, collectively known as "culture change," to make nursing home life feel less institutional. Urged to become safer, nursing homes have undergone an exponential rise in government oversight—only the nuclear power industry is more heavily regulated.

These well-meant responses have not led to better care, however. They have not led to happier, healthier elders, and they have not led to more satisfied families. In fact, the latest efforts to reform nursing homes have had many unintended consequences, some of which have only made matters worse.

In our zeal we have built a *system* of care. The most salient feature of the new regime is the care plan, a written document, which has come to dominate. This document takes precedence over care devised by nursing home doctors, nurses, and other health care professionals, who are given little or no leeway to stray from the institution's charted course of treatment. For those who value freedom and autonomy, the consequences can be dire, not only for the practitioner but most disturbingly for the resident. However inadvertently, it is really the care plan that is served, not the person it is designed to help.

Ironically, the culture change movement has contributed to the trend away from personalized care, at least by people trained to help the elderly and infirm. Intended to make life in a nursing home less institutional, the movement has made it more difficult for nurses, doctors, and other health care professionals to do the jobs they were trained to do to help residents live with some measure of comfort and ease.

Into the vacuum have stepped billing specialists, insurers, lawyers, marketing personnel, and—certainly not least—care plan writers. Such employees influence the shape that long-term care takes. This trend is in keeping with the culture change process, which encourages "equality" among nursing home staff but also leads to misguided or pointless efforts, and sometimes to substandard care for residents.

Within the care plan construct, beliefs and attitudes continue to affect how the old and infirm live out their days. The prevailing philosophy is not so much to respond to actual need but to adhere to a belief system of how care *should* be. As we all know, theory and practice can be quite discordant.

In my earlier book, *Living and Dying in a Long-Term Care Facility: Notes From a Nursing Home Doctor,* I presented individual portraits of some of the many thousands of patients that I have attended over the last decade. Their stories highlighted the problems and predicaments of old age and chronic illness, some of which can be solved and some of which cannot. In this, my latest, book, I examine in greater detail the relationship between residents and staff, within the web we have woven, to show the impacts that our prevailing thinking has on long-term care. The individuals introduced in these pages are actual people that I have met over the course of my professional life. A few are composites, based on more than one of my colleagues or patients. Even when blended, they portray accurately how people work and reside at nursing homes today. To protect privacy, I have used pseudonyms throughout. Conversations quoted in these pages are faithful to true encounters, although I draw on memory and paraphrase them here.

One of my strongest motivations for becoming a doctor was to help other people—and, of course, to do no harm, the physician's first commandment. Yet, over the years that I have been in practice, I have seen the treatment of geriatric syndromes, and the provision of both hospice and palliative care, become subservient to institutional needs.

Sadly, the person for whom a care plan is drawn up fades into a nonentity. At times, it takes a good stretch of the imagination to recognize that there is a person on the other end of the care plan at all. Am I doing no harm now?

I will tell my stories, pose questions, and let readers form their own opinions.

Gilah Silber, M.D.
December 2009

One
Christmas Comes Too Often

The bedside clock reads three in the morning when I am awakened by the ringing telephone. Sally Ballard has expired. She has no vital signs—no pulse, blood pressure, or respirations, the nurse tells me.

"Dr. Silber, can I release the body?"

To get my permission is why Sally's nurse has called me in the middle of the night.

Ordinarily I would offer my stock response to staff I know well in such situations: "Can I tell over the phone that she's dead better than you can tell in person?"

But I am too dazed to joke. The abruptness of Sally's death comes as a surprise, even though she was 101 years old. Only recently did she exhibit mild signs of dementia, and she remained highly mobile.

Sally had been my patient for several years, although she was quick to remind me, "I've lived my whole life without a physician, doc. I don't need one now."

For a centenarian, she was indeed in excellent health but for her high blood pressure. The medicines I gave her to control it made her urinate too much, and she would not take them.

"Dr. Silber, I piss too much already, and I'm not going around in a diaper."

Likewise, she liked salty foods and was not going to give them up, either.

What Sally did need was someone to talk to, and I was as good a person as any. She often engaged me in stories, some of which were about nursing home care gone awry. If she had no use for a medical exam, she always did give me a thorough going-over. She put on her glasses, told me to sit, stand, and then turn around. She loved my clothes. When would she get to wear them? I once heard from a staff member that she would call her daughter after I visited to describe the outfit I had worn. I was gratified. Sally's appreciation for a well-cut suit or a pretty blouse made me realize that I could give some residents, who never left the institution, a little inadvertent sensory pleasure if I simply made a point to dress well when I made my rounds.

Sally also penned a few of her thoughts on a piece of paper and handed them to me some years back. Her poem, "God Has A Risk Manager," inspired me to write my first book, just as it continues to inspire me to tell my—our—story about what it is like to live and die in a long-term care facility. In Sally's poem I read some of my own concerns as a physician in long-term care. In second-guessing illness and aging, sometimes we expend our energy to combat what we cannot change. Too often we forget to behave with compassion and humility when we offer care—the very things that really can make a difference.

I saw Sally for the last time about two weeks before her death. We had our usual chat. Still full of life, she roamed the nursing home corridors in her wheelchair, hounding everyone she met for her cousin's telephone number. I stopped documenting charts long enough to hand her a slip of paper with a number written on it.

"Thank you, Dr. Silber," she said. "You're the only one that helps me."

Not so. Many people attended to Sally. Yet how she saw things was the truth for her, just as it is for the rest of us; "reality" is how we see the moment. The facility was decorating for a Valentine's Day Party, but Sally had her own take on the holiday.

"I can't believe it's Christmas again," she told me. "I liked it better when December came only once a year!"

A nurse whispered to me, "Does Sally need to be put on the psychiatrist's list for this month?"

Out of respect, I pretended not to hear. I doubt that the nurse really wanted an answer, anyway.

Before Day Breaks

At four-thirty, my eyes open again. Sally's words about the blur and acceleration of time have stayed with me for good reason. Often I awake not much more rested than when I went to sleep the night before. When I am on call, I start Monday before Sunday ends, and I end Monday after Tuesday begins. Every week, Sunday is shorter and Monday longer. Is time redefined? If so, I suppose December does now come more than once a year—perhaps twice or three times.

My body is asleep, but my mind is organizing my thoughts and racing through the day. Despite my experience, and a largely repetitive job, there is always some challenge to undertake. At the very least, there is the challenge to maintain enough stamina to care for everyone's needs and to keep my cool.

By the end of the day, I will have traveled more than 120 miles to visit about fifty patients at several nursing homes in the sprawling metropolitan area in which I live. These patients are my "customers" or "clients." I need to satisfy them, not just care for them. I am their employee, after all. There are plenty of doctors in town, and I am certainly not indispensable.

Most of my driving time I will spend on the phone, responding to nursing home staff who need, if not an answer, at least a response. Once I am on-site, staff members will no doubt hound me about something or other as I make my rounds. Residents will follow me like a few ducklings after their mother. Both staff and patients alike will occasionally become irate and imply that I can be blamed—for the plight of the facility, on the one hand, and for the plight of the aging on the other. Ironically, I am also respected and loved.

What keeps me going?

The mere fact that I will return home at night and wake up again in my own bed. No matter where I am or how content to be there, I cannot wait to go home. This love and need I have for my own private space reminds me that these patients of mine have lost precisely that; they can never go home. I cannot turn back their clocks.

Just before five, I get out of bed. It is here in my own home that I am at my most creative during these, the earliest hours of the day, when the excitement of the new meets the mundane and the agony of the old. Luckily, I have not become jaded, a true hazard in the health care professions. If I feel angst, it is because I *do* care. Already a dozen faxes await me in my office off the kitchen. Today I learn that someone has fallen, and that a family member requests that I call her. Then there is the usual stack of routine lab results, pharmacy reviews, and denials of drug coverage for residents. Should I make a substitution that suits their insurance plans? Or should I spend twenty to thirty minutes on the phone to attempt to preauthorize the drug of choice? Will it really make any difference one way or another? It is a financial concern, not a clinical one.

By seven o'clock, I am on the road. I call my mother. She is working on a quilt. I have tried the craft but find it too rigid to be relaxing. Each step depends on the last. One mistake, and everything is ruined. Something in my psyche or training leads me away from such a challenge. Instead I am a multi-tasker. I do jobs in tandem, not necessarily in sequence. Despite its haphazard appearance, everything I do gets done fairly efficiently.

As I start the day, my thoughts go not only to the places that I will visit but also to the people I will see. I will interact not only with my patients but with the people that care for them—the so-called care team. Having practiced medicine in nursing homes for more than a decade, it is pretty easy to anticipate a caregiver's response to a certain situation as well as a patient's. Experience has led me to categorize the care team into six general kinds: normal; bickering (dysfunctional); absent; threatening; passive; and nonexistent. Usually any one team will include overlapping attributes. Sometimes a team will morph altogether from one type to another. In many cases, however, the following characterizations suffice to describe how nursing home staffs function.

The *normal care team* acts as a patient advocate. Its members elicit from residents and their families information that they rely on as part of the decision making regarding care. They take into account each resident's personal choices and act upon them.

The *bickering (dysfunctional) care team* consists of members that hold conflicting opinions regarding residential care. Members of such a team often transmit incomplete or contradictory information to each other. Because no one staff person serves as a point of contact, health care information is in turn relayed in a disjointed manner to residents and their families, who often misinterpret its meaning. Family members and residents consequently become confused, angry, and frustrated.

The *absent care team* generally is unavailable to the resident and resident's family. Its members are preoccupied with interactions among themselves. The team is largely involved in managing the facility and does not focus much attention on the care of residents.

The *threatening care team* bullies residents and their families into accepting staff decisions and facility policy with which they disagree. The team may issue warnings, such as eviction from the nursing home, should residents and their families continue to resist.

The *passive care team* is a cross between the absent and the threatening teams. Members are often difficult to contact but become irate and abusive once they do learn of a situation or issue about which they were not informed. Occasionally members of such a team will interact closely with a few favored residents. Often such a team is composed of a core group that has worked at the facility for a long time, as well as several satellite groups that work in the facility only for a short time.

The *nonexistent care team* is the consequence of a staff whose members constantly come and go. Some are hired by the facility from an outside agency and may only be in the building once or twice a month. Regular staff turnover, even among administrative staff and nurses, is high. Communication between members of such a care team also is nonexistent.

Plans and Puzzles

For every nursing home staff, a large part of the job is to help devise and carry out a care plan to document, problem-solve, and provide care for each resident. Such a plan is also maintained as a record to "prove" adequate care to insurers, the state, and each resident's family.

Just as there are general types of care teams, so, too, are there several types of care plans: There are ones that respond in real time, ones that are retrospective, and still others that are prospective.

The *real time care plan* is made in a progressive manner, rather like a quilt. As a problem arises, a plan is constructed.

The *retrospective care plan* is developed responsively and written after a problem is found; it reminds me of a scrapbook, something

I enjoy making for my own family and as a way to relax and unwind in my free time.

The ***prospective care plan*** is one in which potential problems are arranged like puzzle pieces and their solutions given shape before any actual problem occurs. This "proactive" approach is in vogue at the moment among long-term care administrators. The scripted care plan has become the "art" of medicine, although some of us see it as merely "politically correct" and not particularly useful, as will become clear as I recall some of my experiences.

Whatever its kind, the care plan is a blueprint intended to help the nursing home fulfill its charge to care for its residents. Yet somehow this intention has led not so much to plans as to rules taken at face value and accepted without question. No mere mapping device, the care plan actually leads us into an inverted world: How a resident feels matters less than what the document says he or she is *supposed* to feel. Nor is there always a correlation between the plan and what happens to the resident it was designed to serve. Do cause and effect decouple? Yes, often they do.

As care is systematized, it gets formulated in advance, that is, prepackaged, which can tempt some into deception. It is not unheard of for a nursing home to invent among its residents certain problems that then are neatly solved by the facility's plan of care. The institution can then go on to tout the happy outcome as a tribute to the plan's effectiveness.

As I try to illustrate how care teams and care plans affect life in the nursing home, I am reminded of how my seven-year-old daughter and I put together a jigsaw puzzle. We have become quite the experts and work as a team, sorting and piecing. We started out when she was a preschooler with hundred-piece puzzles; now a thousand-piece one is a cinch. By now it is clear that we can put any puzzle together, regardless of its size. Our ability arises from the successful strategy that we have developed—not to solve any given puzzle in particular—but to complete the construction process. Although we are champions, I wonder. Have we lost something?

In the nursing home, those of us who make up a care team do something similar. We sort through each resident's array of illnesses and various behaviors and conditions, which can be thought of as the pieces of the person's puzzle. In response to each, we assign a strategy. In Sally Ballard's case, for example, we had some success in making her life more comfortable. Only the puzzle we put together never amounted to more than its pieces. We never did understand Sally as a whole person.

Care Takes a Back Seat

Shortly before her death, Sally showed her true colors. In pink nail polish, she painted her SOS signal on the door to the facility's new wing:

"Get me out of here! They're all crazy."

Afterward, she scooted through the front doors of the facility and landed her wheelchair in the mud. A passerby found her quite promptly.

Sally was cleaned up and brought back to her room. Of course, the administrator, the director of nursing, and corporate risk manager were called. So was I, as the facility's medical director. Per guidelines, we had to report the incident to the state. Sally had escaped, and we were supposed to protect her. What if we were sued?

We had, however, a more pressing concern. In less than forty-eight hours, facility board members were due to arrive to celebrate the prized new wing. What were we to do about the front door, with its scrawl of graffiti in pink?

The construction foreman said nail polish was nearly impossible to remove from the sort of material used for the door. We might need to order and install a new one, tasks that could not be accomplished before the wing's official opening. The situation did not look good, at least not until one of the recreational aides created a welcome sign to cover Sally's tracks.

As if embarrassed by all the commotion, Sally laid low. In the days that followed the successful inauguration of the new wing, she ate rarely, slept often, and had little to say for herself. Within a few days, she died peacefully in her sleep.

The rules of the game had ensured that Sally had received plenty of management and documentation but little actual care and concern. Her life and my job were governed by her care plan.

Striving for a gold standard in long-term care is not necessarily a bad idea, although inevitably it will lead to some inflexibility that might be harmful. The problem, however, is that, in reality, there is no gold standard. A care plan supplants real care, rather than upholds it. Based on conventions that become policy and, subsequently, dogma, the plan takes on a life of its own. Its dictates need not be supported by the facts on the ground, even when a plan is adjusted to refine how a resident's life is to be managed. Often, the refinements serve to hide the fact that the plan rests on assumptions that are false to begin with.

What Sally Needed

At 101 years of age, Sally Ballard did not need me to assess her blood pressure a few weeks ago. Sally needed a care *giver*—not a case manager, nor a care plan writer.

Outside the scientific medical model, my heart knew what she really wanted—to say goodbye. Yet I did document her "perfect" blood pressure. Because what if my chart was audited later? Her blood pressure parameter was all that would be evaluated, not whether or not Sally benefited from her farewell conversation with me. If her blood pressure was too high, I might have been paid less. If it continued to be elevated, the insurance company might have placed me on probation. Yet I was not willing to surrender completely to worries about what the insurance company might think. I did not, for example, put this 101-year-old woman on a low-salt diet. The insurance company did not realize that Sally's only joy left in life was a few pretzels and a beer at night while she watched the baseball game.

But I knew.

So I allowed Sally her salted pretzels.

Still, I was careful to document my rationale. I cannot say that I was happy as I did so, but I am, after all, a key player in the game.

The Team Factor

To carry out each care plan, staff members see themselves as a "care team." They also present themselves as a surrogate family, which can cut both ways. Sometimes a team's omnipotence will disrupt the relationship that a resident has with his or her own personal family. Conversely, a team's aloofness can lead to care that is indifferent and to lives led in isolation. As medical and other professional staff play a lesser role in highly regulated facilities, administrative staff with no medical background help define residential care. Often, they have a strong say, and influence standards of practice, or medical protocol.

Unquestionably, the dynamics among team members influence how care plans are executed and carried out. Their personal experience also influences how they respond to each resident's struggle with aging, illness, and death. As we will see, however, experience, even of a professional nature, is no substitute for personal integrity and insight.

Nursing Home Nomad

As soon as Sally Ballard passed away, Betsy Warner arrived to "book" Sally's old room. Betsy was eighty-two. Wheelchair-bound, she had advanced Parkinson's disease, but her mind was clear. She had lived with one of her daughters for about five years until everyone agreed she should enter long-term care. Mother and daughters together had looked at a few facilities before choosing Mission Hill.

Initially, Betsy appeared to adjust well to the facility. She made friends, went to the dining room for meals, and was active socially. In relatively good health, she had no obvious medical problems beyond the Parkinson's. About two months after her arrival, however, she began to complain of symptoms that came and went, mysteriously. At the onset of these bouts, Betsy would take to her bed and telephone her daughters to say that she feared for her life. She insinuated mistreatment at the hands of the staff. Her daughters would come and take her to the emergency room. As these episodes mounted, so did the number of medical specialists she saw, and the diagnostic tests she underwent, for what were always vague complaints. Test results were largely unremarkable. Abruptly, Betsy would return to good health as dramatically as she would soon become ill again. Of course the unending cycle wearied her family. They grew impatient and irate with the lack of a diagnosis. Betsy's care team members shared in the frustration. They tried everything they could think of to help, but they found no way to break the cycle.

In less than a year, the Warner family decided that Betsy should leave Mission Hill, despite its reputation for the best care in the area.

Over the following three years, this elderly woman would live in six different facilities. What may seem farfetched was not so unusual. Most nursing home residents stay in place, it is true. Yet more than a handful of my patients have moved from one facility to another. Each time Betsy moved, of course, a new team of people took care of her. Although her health remained stable, and she had more or less the same set of problems wherever she went, the care she received varied, sometimes significantly, as did her sense of well-being. I bring up Betsy's nomadic behavior here, and elsewhere, because her experience highlights how different care teams function and how striking a difference these variations can make, with consequences that can affect everyone in long-term care, including those that live out their days in but one facility.

Second-Guessing Fate

Every impact has its limits, of course. One realization, which any honest nursing home doctor soon confronts, is that we medical practitioners alter the course of illness and death only at the margins. Family members and patients urge us to combat the natural process. Deep down they know that their demands are unreasonable. Still, they plead with their doctors to find a cure for aging and a way around death. As we will see, however, sometimes fighting the good fight does more harm than good.

Our jobs as doctors is to remain steadfast in our aim to enhance the well-being and longevity of our patients. Eventually, our experience guides us to better understand what is possible and what is not. Yet the urge to second-guess is strong. No doubt many people would be delighted if we gerontologists could hire God Himself as a consultant. Come to think of it, God Himself would do well to hire a consultant to guide Him through the complex maze that is the long-term care industry in America, where good care often is at odds with the competing needs of insurance companies, government, and LTC corporate management, just as it often is at odds with the expectations of families, the abilities of nursing home staff, and even with the desires of residents themselves.

Two
Culture Change Comes to the Sanctuary

The normal care team is a rarity. Of the more than thirty long-term care facilities in which I have practiced medicine, only Mission Hill could be said to maintain one. Again, by "normal" I mean only that the team carries out its functions in the smoothest and most effective ways possible. I do not mean that Mission Hill is the only facility I know of that offers residents good care. Good care is not always normal care. In fact, normal care is not right for everyone, and some residents of Mission Hill do not respond well to the care that is offered there. Normal is not what they need.

As I entered the parking lot one recent morning, I was perturbed by someone on the night staff that did not park properly and took up two parking spaces. I am a perfectionist. I think about standards, which at Mission Hill are set high. I set my standards similarly. Yet I also know that I was lucky to seek out a parking spot in what is a sylvan setting along the river. I can think of another facility, for example, where the lot is so small that I am forced to park across the street at Wal-Mart and dart across lanes of heavy traffic. I also visit a facility in a poor part of town, and went there once when a curfew was still in force after a race riot. I could not put off my need to be there. A patient was critically ill, and his family wanted me at his bedside to discuss what came next.

Postponement of my visits is rarely an option under any circumstances. It would be illegal for me to skip the requisite monthly checkup of any patient in long-term care, even if she or he was in a stable state of health. Does a 101-year-old woman like Sally Ballard, who had no medical problems, need to see me and pay for my specialized services every month? Yes, if she lives in a long-term care facility in the state in which I work.

Sanctuary

Locals call Mission Hill the "Sanctuary," and it lives up to the name. Surely it is the most beautiful facility I visit, given its natural surroundings. Home to about a hundred residents (most of whom are under my care) Mission Hill employs several hundred staff.

If my own family could not care for me, I would choose to live here. I am proud to be a team member. A few of the staff are soul mates. Others I do not know as well, but we are all still friends. We work together like a family, although sometimes a cranky one.

At the time of the visit I record here, Mission Hill was in the throes of major changes, both physical and philosophical. The old building was undergoing renovation. Small, semi-private rooms were expanding into large, completely private ones, with large windows to overlook pristine wetlands. I was delighted by the improvements, but I worried too. How would the residents react to the transformation? All of the paintings had been taken down, for one thing. For years, familiar pictures had hung in the corridors, and served as landmarks as much as they did decor. Even the public restroom off the lobby had disappeared. If I was disoriented, how must the residents have felt?

In tandem with the physical facelift, Mission Hill was poised to adopt an approach to care widely known as "culture change," intended to create a more personal, homelike atmosphere in nursing homes. That description already applied to Mission Hill, as far as most of us were concerned.

To make the change, we staff underwent formal education— for which Mission Hill paid top dollar—to receive accreditation as a person-centered, long-term care community. As part of the process, which took years to complete, Mission Hill pledged to run a facility that supports autonomy, diversity, and individual choice, as well as responsiveness, spontaneity, and continuous learning and growth. Residents were to participate in everyday decisions regarding their care, and their families were to be seen in partnership with residents and staff.

Among other things, on paper at least, everyone on staff was an equal now and expected, if not required, to job-share, just as we would have shared chores in a considerate, cooperative household.

Chilly Atmosphere

Among the distinguishing characteristics of a facility with a normal care team is the ability to attract and keep staff. Mission Hill could rightly take pride in maintaining Holly Martin, a capable administrator, for the first twenty-five years of operation. Stability of that kind is exceedingly rare in nursing homes. Far more typical is to watch as one administrator is escorted out of the building without warning by the chief of the janitorial staff on Friday, and to welcome a brand new administrator as he or she makes an abrupt first appearance on Monday—a turn of events that plays out like a divorce after a quickie Vegas marriage.

Mission Hill has not featured these kinds of scenes, because it takes the time to hire carefully. In addition to her business acumen, Holly had a warm, friendly personality and made it a point to know the residents, their families, as well as all members of the staff. When it came time for her to think about retirement, Holly made all the right moves. Over the course of a year, she interviewed many candidates to fill her job. When she announced her handpicked successor, she was able to recommend Brenda Talbot without reservation and to offer her personal stamp of approval. Holly's approval meant a lot to the staff, because it reflected the successful completion of the mentorship that Brenda had received over the past four months. Holly taught her soon-to-be successor about the business aspects of Mission Hill, as well as about its staff dynamics, resident culture, and facility customs and practices. She introduced Brenda to each of the residents and made sure she was thoroughly familiar with the entire facility.

Once settled in, Brenda turned out to be a brilliant business administrator, quick to solve problems and settle disputes as part of the day-to-day management of the facility. She kept corporate headquarters happy, too, by maintaining a strong, positive cash flow.

Although she embraced the bottom line, she embraced little else, however.

What Holly had not been able to teach Brenda was how to love the residents. Brenda was chilly toward staff too. In a word she considered them replaceable, no matter how talented and skilled. This absence of affection could be felt in the atmosphere. The coolness filtered down until eventually it spread through every aspect of care, dampening the enthusiasm with which care was delivered, even though Mission Hill had by then earned its accreditation as an official culture change facility.

Yet because business skills are so crucial to running nursing homes, Brenda's abilities have made her a fine nursing home administrator in the eyes of her corporate employers. Thus far, she appears willing to stay and offer the benefit of long-term stewardship, which Mission Hill has always enjoyed. Residents and staff alike, however, consider her not quite up to the "Holly" Grail. Although it is true that Brenda could probably run a major corporation, in fact, she is in charge of frail, vulnerable, dying people. Her decisions affect the rest of their short lives.

Disaffection and a Dog

Sometimes a change in staff can have a domino effect and lead to a flurry of comings and goings. That did not happen at Mission Hill, probably because the staff was a well-knit one, and most of its members had served there a long time. Like Holly, Ingrid Ekstrom had held her position since the facility's inception. She stayed on as director of nursing, despite Brenda's sharper-edged management style. After so many years of service, Ingrid was well integrated into the Mission Hill environment. She adhered to corporate policy, and loved and served the residents at the same time. Truth be told, however, she was in dire financial straits and depended on her job, despite the fact that she was near retirement age.

As day nursing supervisor, Lydia Howard stayed on as well. She had started her career as a nursing assistant years ago. The facility had helped pay for her further education, and in time she became a registered nurse. Mission Hill had become her true family. Long ago, Ingrid had taken Lydia under her wing and assumed the role of surrogate mother. Holly had been her "grandmother." Perhaps I was her "sister." An only child, I certainly saw Lydia as mine.

It did not surprise me when she began to show signs of decline in mood and morale, however. The absence of Holly, who had run Mission Hill with such familial warmth and with whom Lydia had had such strong emotional ties, was bound to cause a sense of loss. Brenda offered little emotional compensation. Beyond these disappointments was Lydia's dislike of everything to do with culture change.

"They don't need me anymore," she told me one day. "All that training is defunct," by which she meant training to make complex nursing decisions. Once Mission Hill adopted culture change, staff were expected to defer more than ever to state mandates on what to do and when to do it. Lydia felt like she was on automatic pilot. Other staff members were beginning to feel the same way, she sensed, and the quality of care may have fallen off as a result.

"Maybe it has," I told her, "but, trust me, it's still good care." Lydia had never worked anywhere else, so she had no idea how bad things really could be.

The one exception to Lydia's dislike of culture change was Bella, a Golden Labrador Retriever.

Culture change encourages the introduction of a cat or a dog into the facility, and Bella was the mascot of the movement at Mission Hill. To make herself useful, Lydia groomed the dog and took her for long walks on the paths that ran through Mission Hills's surrounding wetlands.

Bella did not remain at Mission Hill for long. She soon went to live as a companion to a former resident, who had gone into hospice care at home. The man's family members were better equipped than the nursing home staff to care for a good-sized dog like Bella, with her need for a daily routine that included outdoor exercise. Bella's short stay was a sad development for those who had grown fond of her, but it was an unsurprising one, given the nursing home environment, which was not ideal for a dog. Like the other residents, Bella was expected to live in a somewhat structured manner, attuned to modern heath care management and federal regulation, culture change notwithstanding. Nursing home rules are based on certain conventions not easily learned by an animal. Bella could not understand and follow rules that had nothing to do with food, approval, or other physical or primal emotions.

Bella's departure affected Lydia deeply. She grew more listless in the weeks that followed. Of course she still cared about her job, just not as much. If a mistake was made, it was not quite as important as it used to be. Work got done during the day but at a slower pace. Fine points, which she used to deem essential, were not critical anymore. In a word, Lydia was no longer conscientious, much to my dismay. Brenda never noticed. She had not administered Mission Hill long enough to know Lydia well. More important, culture change and her own nature led her to pay less attention to the ups and downs of individual staff members. The warm and friendly exchanges that used to occur between Holly and Lydia were a thing of the past. Now when the brisk new administrator and the despondent day supervisor of nurses passed each other in the hall, they did so without acknowledgment, as if each were a figment of the other's imagination.

Even though Lydia no longer loved her job, she feared she might lose it. By that time, the facility's remodeling was well under way, and nowhere in the plans was it shown where her office would be relocated. I tried to reassure her. We were all going through upheaval but would soon adjust. Most of the difficulties would resolve themselves. I could see that she remained unconvinced.

In fact, Lydia was able to rally some staff into joining her in rejection of culture change. The consequences, however, were counterproductive. A few of the better nurses did leave Mission Hill in protest, but their absence only affected the residents—not the "movement." Lydia won the battle but lost the war. Brushing aside resident care and staff concerns, culture change advocates pressed forward, in full swing, leaving doubters and naysayers in the dust.

No Stand on Ceremony

Lydia's counterpart in the evening took quite a different attitude toward the recent change in operating policy. Carol Sue Redmon was unfazed, probably because she did not *believe* strongly in the modern practice of medicine. I stress the word "believe," because medicine is not entirely a science. Often it is just that—a belief system. She was, however, a strong believer in caring, in a job well done, and in the judicious use of facts.

Sixty and somewhat overweight, Carol Sue had severe hip osteoarthritis, which caused her to hobble about the facility. She knew she was aging and her health was not great, but she also knew that there was not much that she could do about it. No doubt her tendency to make the best of her own situation carried over into her attitude on the job.

Although she held a supervisory position, she was not one to stand on ceremony. If something needed to be done, she would do it, no matter how menial or out of the realm of her job description. This attitude was much in keeping with culture change, which embodies a strong, egalitarian work ethic.

Yet Carol Sue did not really like culture change. It was just that she knew from years of working with the elderly that, once she stopped being active, a quick decline in her own health might proceed. Carol Sue was not ready to give up her job but neither would she need to look for a new one. Her family's financial status was strong. So she felt free to express dissatisfaction with facility policies. She boycotted senseless meetings and made snide remarks about those whose professional conduct she did not find up to par. If she was fired as a consequence, or her job was made more difficult, she could leave without repercussion.

I depended on her offbeat humor. When I called her during her night shifts, she would entertain me with one of her signature sayings: "I'm cooking on a front burner tonight, Gilah." Or "That new little gal on the first floor is a couple sandwiches short of a picnic." Above all, I prized her generally sunny outlook. As she might say, "I'm as happy as a clam at high tide." Carol Sue was irreplaceable. She could not be matched—although some would like her to be—by an ace care plan writer.

Culture and Career Change

Such an ace would be Zoë Wright. In her mid-forties, Zoë had an advanced nursing degree and had spent most of her career in academic nursing, mostly teaching. Although highly skilled, she had little experience in direct patient care. After her divorce and her last child left home for college, however, she felt in need of a change. She came to Mission Hill to serve as a minimum data set (MDS) nurse. Zoë's career path may have altered, but she continued to work in a rather aloof fashion and did not get to know the residents. She took charts, went to her office, researched them, and produced the MDS, a rather lengthy document mandated by the federal government, filled out on each resident at least quarterly, and better known as a care plan.

Zoë was not well liked by the other team members. They viewed her plans as a hindrance more than a help as they attended to the residents. Moreover, as Lydia noticed, culture change led Mission Hill to focus on adherence to state mandates more and more and to favor reliance on any one nurse's knowledge and skills less and less. Thus, as administration and corporate tacitly made known, Zoë's skills as a care plan writer met with more approval than, say, Carol Sue's or Lydia's as nursing supervisors.

Staff members that worked closely with the residents were less likely to embrace culture change. A floor nurse like Kathy Catanzaro was a perfect example. She had given direct care to the residents every working day for twenty-some years. Her job was hard, but she had always loved it. Now, in just a few short months, everything had changed. How did it happen so quickly, she wondered. The process of aging and dying had not changed much, she said. It was the business and management of aging and dying that had.

At first Kathy assumed decades of experience would help her cope with culture change. Native to the surrounding metropolis, she had known many of the residents and their extended families since childhood. Everyone trusted her.

One morning when I was making my rounds, Kathy called out to me from the new dining area to say hello. It took me a moment to recognize her. Wearing a hairnet and oversized rubber gloves, she was in the process of pushing a large dumpster of trash toward the kitchen, not the job of a nurse as far as I knew. I had just come away from a patient that had recently undergone surgery, who told me he had asked several times for a pain medication; he was quite angry because he was not being helped. Little did he know that his floor nurse was otherwise engaged, busy taking out the trash as part of the new regime.

Culture change at Mission Hill entailed giving up fixed roles and being willing to share new duties. Soon Kathy would help the nutritional aides feed the residents their breakfast. Then she would walk Bella, who was still in residence at the time. Later, she would cover for the receptionist. No one, however, would help *her* take care of resident wounds or give residents their medicines. The receptionist and kitchen aides simply did not have the training to do so. These facts went unmentioned.

"Care to give me a hand?" Kathy joked, pointing at the dumpster. "Better yet, walk that damned dog for me today, okay? There's a clause in your contract, don't forget, doc. You know the one—something about doing whatever 'duties' are 'deemed necessary.'"

I supposed that there was.

Kathy was practical, kind, and down to earth. She was also intelligent and certainly could have pursued her education to become an advanced practice nurse. She preferred her job as a floor nurse and her direct involvement in the lives of her patients. She had no interest in writing care plans or working in administration. All of her qualities did help her persevere for some time.

On a particularly bad day, however, she confided in me. "You know, Gilah, sometimes I think I'd be better off as a barmaid. I'd still be in a helping profession, if you know what I mean. I'd be listening to people's woes and giving them advice. Only I wouldn't have to follow so many rules and fill out so many forms."

She had my sympathy regarding the rules and forms. "We need you here, though, Kathy. Your nursing skills are first-rate. You're part of why Mission Hill offers excellent care."

Kathy disagreed. "We're going downhill, I'd say. Culture change was supposed to make this place more like home. Instead, we've got the worst of both worlds. Now I get to be a janitor and a dog-walker, as well as a nurse. There's no letup on the red tape. I still have to document every move I make."

Kathy and I held many impromptu discussions over the next few months. I continued to remind her how much she contributed to the lives of her friends at Mission Hill. Ultimately, however, Kathy decided to leave the facility. She did go on to become a barmaid, a career move that turned out much as she predicted. Patrons tipped her extra, thanks to her keen ability to listen. Alas, Kathy's superb abilities to nurse went to waste.

"They were starting to go to waste at Mission Hill, too," she said.

Culture Change and Clout

The great leveling meant a boost in clout among those eager to flex more muscle. With its emphasis on egalitarianism, culture change brought out latent tendencies at Mission Hill, including certain conceits. Such was the case with Cammie Faust, the retired beautician that came to the facility several times a week. Close in age to many of the women in residence, she and they had long ago developed a strong rapport as she styled their hair. Many women saw Cammie at least once a week for an hour, which was certainly more time than they spent with me, their physician. She in turn offered them advice—not that it always was sound. This detail seemed to elude some of the ladies that greatly enjoyed Cammie's services—and took whatever she said to heart. For better and for worse, she wielded influence, something that culture change, with its blurring of hierarchy and position titles, tended to inflate.

In the past, I avoided Cammie's lair and sent a nurse in my stead, should, God forbid, I need to see a patient while she was still under the beautician's care. The few times that I entered the salon myself, I got a frosty reception. Cammie met my request to see her clients only grudgingly. I am not implying that I am more important than Cammie. I am a firm believer that every human being is to be treated with equal respect. We do serve different needs and purposes, however, which cannot always go unrecognized. At Mission Hill, I was a specialized consultant. Because I was in the facility for such a short time, I would have appreciated it if Cammie could have viewed medical appointments as her customers' first priority.

Cammie was not inclined to see things my way. She loved the metamorphosis at Mission Hill. At last, the institution appeared to give her services as much or more priority than mine. If I needed to see a patient who was having her hair done, I would have to wait until Cammie had finished.

Of course Cammie would have been the first to admit that she was not a doctor or a nurse, but as culture change took hold, she grew more boldly confident and assertive as she advised residents on dilemmas such as whether or not to stay on certain medications, or whether to opt for surgery. A case in point involved Alma Smith, one of my oldest patients and very much in Cammie's thrall. Alma developed a case of hemorrhoids, and Cammie decided that she would cure her. She brought in newspaper articles, advertisements, and every bit of information that she could find about hemorrhoids. These she passed on to Alma, confidentially, when she washed and set her hair. Carol Sue got wind of a certain advertisement one day. She confiscated it, believing it to be a scam.

I tended to agree but returned the advertisement to Alma.

"I'm skeptical that the advertised process will help you," I told her, "and insurance won't cover something that experimental. Still, if you do want to pursue it, let's find out everything we can and talk about it some more."

"Okay," Alma said. "That sounds like a good idea."

Cammie, in her beauty salon/outpatient surgery center, however, had other ideas. What Alma really needed to do was to change physicians. This, in fact, was what she did.

Why did Alma take her hairstylist's advice, when plenty of medically informed counsel was available? I recall an experience I had with my younger daughter.

Waiting for Santa

When she was seven, Avishav insisted on going to see Santa Claus. I knew she did not really believe in him anymore, but she continued to try to, despite overwhelming evidence to the contrary. Her two older siblings had debunked him openly, and she was being raised in a family of heretical Jews. In her attempt to hang on to her shaky conviction, she no longer asked questions out of innocent curiosity—"How can he be at the mall and the zoo at the same time, Mom?" Now she was afraid of the answer.

Unbelievers, though we may be, we are a kind family. Patiently we waited in the long line at the mall with Avishav—father, mother, and teenage sister and brother. I looked at the crowd around us—physicians, attorneys, laborers, and salesmen. I doubted that anyone but the youngest in line actually believed that Santa was real, although we politely upheld the pretense. There was no enjoyment in the process, it cost money, and nothing was really gained in the end. We were taking time from our precious weekend to engage in make-believe. Why, I wondered, were we all here? If we stopped bringing children to see Santa, would we have to give up on our own grownup hopes and dreams as well?

My friend Robin let her daughter, Sarah, see Santa when she was younger yet gently told her that he was not real, only part of the celebration. Many years later, a Girl Scout troop leader called to complain that Sarah had upset the other girls, because she said that Santa was not real. Apparently even at age eleven, her fellow scouts were not ready to give up the fantasy.

Santa and Cammie also bring me back to the care plan. Few of us who work in nursing homes actually believe in the wisdom of such plans to provide our residents with superior care, yet we bow to convention and uphold the pretense. In fact, the care plan is largely a complicated game, to be played, mastered, and won. The expert that writes such plans is not a real caregiver, any more than the old gent at the shopping mall is Santa. At Mission Hill, Zoë Wright could write a stellar plan without ever even laying eyes on a patient.

"Cammie" Change and the Care Plan

As a care plan aficionado, Zoë already was a talented writer. In her zeal to excel, however, she took classes to learn how to write great plans, and then wrote and rewrote to perfection the ones that she produced on the job. She knew the state regulations inside out, and all the loopholes and ways to avoid difficult issues. Her reputation grew beyond Mission Hill. Competitors sought her out regularly with offers of hefty salary increases. To Mission Hill's credit, she turned them down. Given her inventiveness, she probably would have made a good novelist. Although she wrote each individual plan, she never met a resident in person but worked off names and diagnoses only. She had little use for people and treated the residents the same way she treated everyone else, that is, with a bit of arrogance and disdain. Proud of all her plans, Zoë took particular satisfaction in the one that involved "Tiki," a Calico kitten.

After Bella left the facility, Mission Hill introduced another animal—this time a cat—in keeping with the homelike atmosphere that culture change encourages. A cat, it was hoped, would require less time and attention from the staff than had a dog. Most of the residents loved "Tiki." Something fresh among old, withered bodies, she gave love and affection and was a sign of life. As was to be expected, a few did not like the cat. One of them decided to complain; or rather her daughter did, on her behalf.

Daughter took Mother's complaint straight to the top. She bypassed both the administrator and the director of nursing, and instead put in a call to the state ombudsman. The daughter's plan of attack no doubt reflected the fact that Mission Hill had recently sent her mother a thirty-day notice of eviction; her bill for room and board had not been paid for nearly six months. Soon the state initiated a "survey" to deal with the complaint. At "issue" was the source of payment for the cat's upkeep.

Bright one morning, the survey team arrived. They recognized culture change, but rules still applied. In this case, the state concluded that the facility had violated none with regard to the upkeep of the cat (no resident funds were used for the purpose), but other issues arose. The facility was asked to demonstrate that the cat:

1. Did not put either its own health in danger, or that of the elderly and infirm residents among whom it lived;
2. Lived in a safe environment in which all of its physical needs were met; and
3. Did not compromise the dignity of any of the residents with regard, say, to their privacy in the bathroom.

Mission Hill had thirty days to come up with an official plan of action. No problem. The state complaint team and the mother-daughter duo had met their match. Zoë, the care plan writer, loved the cat. She was determined that Tiki would stay on at Mission Hill, if it took her the full thirty days to make her case. Not only would the cat stay, but the facility would also be deficiency-free. Zoë proceeded in a systematic manner. For once, she rallied support. She came down from her pedestal and elicited help from all the experts.

As the medical director, I was asked to ensure that the cat was not a threat to human health. A veterinarian's assessment and documentation were all in order. The cat certainly was in good shape, and she did not harm the residents.

Second, the cat's own physical needs were investigated. Indeed, our cat was given all the care, nutrition, and exercise scientifically recommended for this type of animal. The team had addressed these important issues previously without state interference.

The last and third consideration was more difficult to ensure, dealing as it did with inter-species interactions and how to anticipate what impact they would have on privacy and human dignity.

Zoë went all out on this one. She went straight to the biology department at the regional university. Scientifically, cats do not have complex emotions in line with those of humans. It was not possible for Tiki to "ogle" breasts or other private parts. Just the same, to be on the safe side, Zoë's care plan instructed that the cat not be allowed into any room where a resident was undressing or carrying out personal grooming and hygiene activities. We would go above and beyond the rules—we would make a new one.

How would we document our plan? State regulators were familiar with the use of a resident's chart and care plan for that purpose, so Mission Hill created a chart for Tiki, and staff wrote in it every day to record when the cat ate and what, when it defecated, when it slept, and when it played and exercised. There was even a sign-out sheet, which staff used to record Tiki's whereabouts in the facility at all times. The transfer of data from the cat's chart and signup sheet became still another task for Kathy Catanzaro, who had not yet left Mission Hill.

Zoë's care plan did turn out to be a resounding success. When the state inspectors returned, they found no deficiencies. In fact, they praised the facility for its flawless documentation. Zoë won, and Tiki stayed. Her story did not end there, however.

The Cat Carries On

Betsy Warner, the high-strung and soon-to-be nomadic lady we met earlier, was still in residence at the time. Given her mood swings, it was not surprising that she developed a love-hate relationship with Tiki. One day she insisted on sleeping with the cat; the next day, she complained that Tiki smelled and made her stomach pain worse. The staff grew concerned, especially Zoë, who took pride in Tiki's presence at Mission Hill, a clear sign of the facility's adherence to culture change, and of her own skill as a care plan writer.

Care team members focused hard on Betsy's case during their regular reviews of each resident's care. She had unexplained abdominal pain, unexplained headaches, and unexplained episodes of lethargy. I saw her frequently and ordered multiple tests with numerous specialists, to no avail. The staff and I continued to work with consultants, and to read the literature for possible diagnoses.

Betsy continued to wax and wane. One day she monopolized Tiki; the next she shrieked when the cat approached her. Staff made heroic efforts to anticipate Betsy's moods. Zoë grew quick at swooping in and depositing Tiki into the basket she kept in her office. Even so, Betsy managed to have a showdown with Tiki now and again, which took its toll. The staff grew weary of the need for constant vigilance and occasional intervention. Betsy herself seemed to grow more confused and despondent, as did Tiki.

It began to look as if the cat would have to go after all. Then one day Kathy, who had known Betsy and her family for a long time, stopped me on my rounds to offer some information. Mrs. Warner's youngest daughter had just had a baby. Betsy was joyful at the prospect of her first grandchild but, ever since the baby's arrival six weeks ago, her daughter had not been in to visit.

"I know I'm playing amateur sleuth here," Kathy said to me, "but I wonder if Betsy isn't acting out." In her conflicted behavior toward Tiki, perhaps she was expressing both joy at her grandchild's birth, and jealousy and sadness because she missed seeing her daughter.

Such a thought had not occurred to me. I had been too hard at work in search of a physical or psychiatric cause for Betsy's extreme reactions to the cat.

With the solution in sight, the care team shook off its weariness and leapt into action. Staff arranged a conference with Mrs. Warner's youngest daughter and her husband to explain the lack of diagnoses for Betsy's recent physical complaints, on the one hand, and to convey on the other, her enjoyment of regular visits from family members. The couple was open to the suggestion that Mrs. Warner might be feeling lonelier lately and fearful of abandonment. They agreed to hire a babysitter so that Betsy's youngest child could resume her weekly visits to her mother. Several months later, the whole wing rejoiced when Mrs. Warner's grandchild paid her first visit.

Staff no longer had to dwell on Betsy's case during their care conferences. Her physical complaints had resolved to a significant degree. She had even begun to develop closer relationships with other residents as her emotions grew more stable. Zoë could breathe a sigh of relief as well. Betsy and Tiki were again on the best of terms.

Betsy's story illustrates the advantages of the normal care team. Even as Mission Hill was in the throes of its adjustment to culture change, team members were able to offer consistently good care.

As the facility's medical director, I was proud, of course. Through extraordinary effort the staff had succeeded in keeping on board a beloved pet. Still, the outcome was not good for everyone. The mother and daughter that had complained to the state about Tiki's presence remained unhappy. The anonymity of their complaint had put a personal response out of reach, even by a well-adjusted care team. It saddened me, also, that the wisdom that allowed us to help the distraught Betsy Warner belonged to a wonderful, soon-to-be-ex, floor nurse, Kathy Catanzaro.

All in all, the Tiki episode left me with quite a lot of food for thought. Was professional counseling in order? No, of course not, I had Carol Sue.

Three
Carol Sue and the Rule of Rules

I rarely laid eyes on Carol Sue, who worked the evening shift as nursing supervisor, whereas I made my medical rounds early. Yet the two of us spoke every day, perhaps more than I spoke to my husband and children. When she was arriving for her shift at Mission Hill, I would be in the school parking lot, picking up my children. She would often call me then on my cell phone with questions and for an update. Over time, I associated after-school with Carol Sue. So did my children—Shira, Avishav, and Jared—who long ago grew accustomed to her "stat" calls.

"Has Carol Sue called today?" my son would ask on the way home.

When they heard me laughing over the phone, Shira would ask, "Are you talking to Carol Sue again?"

At home I would pour a glass of wine and then call Carol Sue as I prepared dinner. Our phone conversations became part of my evening routine, and her gifts to me over the years reflected that routine as well—a cookbook that I used often, aptly entitled the *Dinner Doctor*, and the occasional bottle of wine, despite the fact that she was a teetotaler. Ostensibly, I would call to see if she needed anything before the end of the day. In fact, I called because I needed to talk to her. If I did not call her, she would call me about something that probably could have waited until the next day—or the next week. I guess we both had a similar hidden agenda: We needed to vent our frustrations over an increasingly difficult job.

Soul mates, we are hardly two peas in a pod. I am Jewish and a Libertarian, after growing up as a Democrat. She is Catholic and an avid Republican—yet one with the free spirit that reminds me of a California hippie in the nineteen sixties. Some of our differences remain unacknowledged—we love each other too much to let politics and religion interfere. Yet over time, as our friendship has developed, most of what separates us has seemed to dissolve to the point of non-existence. Our conversations heal us, and there is little that we have not discussed. She knows, for example, that I, the "dying expert," fear mortality, and she helped me through a rough patch when I could not sleep, or else I awoke from nightmares about the death of my husband and children.

In turn, I got to know Carol Sue's joys and sorrows, especially those that involved her elderly parents. One mystery that never quite got solved was why she had placed them in Serenity Acres, a facility that offered subpar nursing at near top dollar. Her father had had the moxie to start and then run his own large, successful corpora-tion. His wealth meant that everything was paid for out of pocket, a substantial amount each month, to reside in a place where nursing was not nearly as good as it was at Mission Hill. What was Carol Sue thinking?

Serenity Acres was close to her own home, she explained. "I don't want to work at Mission all day, and then spend my spare time there also. Besides, Mom and Dad aren't sick; they're just old. They don't need specialized care, so it doesn't have to be the best."

Still, I wondered: Could her disdain for culture change out-weigh her low opinion of mediocre nursing care?

In any case, I took her parents on as my patients. Her dad was one of my favorites, although not favored by many. His antics did not bother me. When I first met him, he flatulated, apparently quite de-liberately by way of greeting, and gave me the look of a mischievous child. Many times when I visited him, he would tell me that he had no need of me. Why would he need me? I could not bring back his youth. When his "thanks" finally came, I felt quite touched. Later, I sobbed when Carol Sue called me to pronounce his death. As for her mother, she was a saint in all respects. She ended her days blind and silent.

More than anything, Carol Sue and I learned from each other. From me she learned my favorite quote, one of Friedrich Nietzsche's most memorable: "That which does not kill us makes us stronger."

With that in mind, we figured we were both fitter than Hercules, even though we hardly ever made it to the gym.

What I learned from Carol Sue was the paradox that you could not hope to change the rules unless you followed them to the letter. I did not do that as well as she did. Interestingly, she never let her own opinions interfere. She followed every rule—even the ones she disagreed with openly.

At times her unflagging adherence to every single nursing home regulation put us at odds. I like to think I was her equal in upholding the highest standards. It was that one percent that led to our quibbling—when we both agreed it was absurd to follow a rule in the given context. I would urge her to see reason rather than rules as paramount. She never conceded.

"We'll end up in the clink," she would warn, if we did not do what we were supposed to do.

No Cough Drop, No Clink

There was the time, for example, when a short-term resident wanted to keep a box of cough drops at her bedside. The patient was alert and healthy and had come to Mission Hill for rehabilitation after an elective hip replacement. Yet her simple request was not easily met. Carol Sue would have had to call a facility nurse every thirty minutes to administer the sugary lozenge, purchased at the checkout of the local grocery. To do otherwise would violate guidelines that prohibited residents from having *any* type of medication in their possession. At one time, such rules applied to prescription medications only. Gradually, however, their reach has extended to anything that conceivably could be viewed as medicinal, including over-the-counter cough drops, lip balms, and lotions for dry skin. Intended to protect the patient from overdose or other misuse of a physician's prescription, such rules have been taken to extreme. In their extreme form, they are frequently overlooked. Not at Mission Hill, however, at least not on Carol Sue's watch. A rule is a rule is a rule, and it must be followed, though she could be tongue-in-cheek:

"If we leave the woman alone with the cough drops," she told me, "she'll choke on one. The minute she does, state inspectors will show up and close us down."

All joking aside, however, she refused to allow me to authorize the box of cough drops at bedside.

Rules With an Attitude

Carol Sue and most of the staff at Mission Hill tried to believe in pointless rules, just as my daughter tried to believe in Santa. This strict adherence sets Mission Hill apart from other nursing homes. Perhaps it may seem ironic that this nursing home, with its rare, normal care team, is the one that actually dots every dot and crosses every tee, no matter how trivial. The way Carol Sue and most of her colleagues see it, however, noncompliance would not make things better; the trivial rules would not disappear. Were a staff member to ignore the trivia, it would only make him or her look sloppy, and unprofessional. Despite my own exasperation at times, I must concede that I can see the wisdom in such an attitude, especially when I see what happens elsewhere.

Elsewhere, staff do resist rules that have little or no meaning. They seek ways to evade them and still look compliant. The more such an attitude prevails, in my experience, the more long-term staff take on the disgruntled characteristics of a bickering care team. Sometimes dissatisfaction provides the impetus for a coup and the adoption of a whole new set of internal rules. Sometimes the new rules are worse, anchored as they are to the flimsy pedestal of the old.

All in all, when it comes to the status quo, two basic nursing home rules would seem to apply, although they may at times appear contradictory:

Rule 1. If there is a rule, it must be followed.

Rule 2. Rules must be relatively equal in weight or value. If not, there are too many rules.

Experience also inspires me to recommend some new rules regarding rules:

Rule 1. Rules can be re-evaluated.

Rule 2. To solve a new problem does not necessarily mean that we must create a new rule.

These recommendations of mine are more ambitious than they might seem. The stories that I recount in the rest of this chapter begin to show why.

Doorbell Protocol

The physical remodeling that Mission Hill underwent to adapt to culture change created an opportune time to add on a dementia, or "special care," unit to provide high-quality Alzheimer and behavioral management. The unit was carefully thought-out as to décor and physical layout, eating arrangements, personal and medical care, and safety. As is typical of such units, the door would remain locked, and visitors would use a security code to enter. A doorbell also was placed on the outside of the unit for those that did not know the code.

Somehow, of all of the potential issues that might have arisen to cause difficulties in the new dementia unit, friction centered on the doorbell. Disputes arose about who would have to answer the bell and when precisely the bell would be used. During planning meetings, staff drifted away from the agenda to return to these questions, but not many were resolved.

Things came to a head when the psychiatrist Edgar Berning arrived to make his monthly rounds. Dr. Berning had had patients at Mission Hill for many years. He was known for his kindness, even temperament, and for his shyness. He took a conservative and realistic approach to his patients and was sought-after throughout the interstate area.

He had many residents to see in the new dementia unit but did not know the security code, which at that point was restricted to day staff. He rang the bell. Five or so minutes passed, and no one answered. He rang again, and again got no response. Knowing the rest of the facility well, Dr. Berning found the director of nursing, who let him into the unit.

Once inside, he was confronted by Valerie, the dementia unit manager.

"Was that you out there, ringing the bell? What a headache you're giving everybody."

"Well, give me the code to the door, and I won't be a bother in future," the doctor said.

Valerie's reply was sharp. "Not unless you guarantee that none of my residents will wander."

"Valerie, I'm offended. If I were God, as you seem to be asking me to be, would I have to ring the bell?"

Valerie might have laughed, but she was not really paying attention to Dr. Berning's actual words. She was a lady on a mission, and her mission was to control the door.

"You'll just have to wait for the bell like everybody else," she said. "Nobody gets special service around here anymore."

"We may all be equal, but we're not all the same," the doctor replied. "Some of us learn from our mistakes and others don't."

Mission Hill lost a psychiatrist that day but retained a doorbell. The standing committee that dealt with the dementia unit did, however, recommend a new protocol on how to use it: Visitors would now be asked to ring the doorbell at least five times—and wait at least two minutes between each ring—before they sought assistance from administration to enter the dementia unit. Thus visitors could wait as much as ten minutes outside the door. The bottom line: We provided a doorbell but not necessarily anyone to answer it. No rule, after all, said that someone had to be on hand to do that. Not yet, anyway.

Clearly rules arise to settle internal conflicts, and may be seen as the only way that problems can be solved, even simple collisions, such as the one between the nursing supervisor and the psychiatrist over the doorbell. Their skirmish might have led to something simple, like playground rules in elementary school. Instead, the resolution was not a helpful one, and discourteous to visitors.

The Cranberry Juice Rule

Ironically, Mission Hill's aim for perfection made it prey to more regulation, when state inspectors found fault only in the undocumented change in a glass of juice. Final outcome: New fine print to heed on the breakfast tray. Here is how it happened.

Typically, Mission Hill comes up deficiency-free in state surveys. Although actual care is excellent, the good "grades" are mainly the result of impeccable care plans. After a few years of "too many" perfect surveys, the state was rumored to have created a set of "new rules," which it applied only to Mission Hill.

How had the rumor become the latest gossip? The facility down the street was not good. In its last survey, the state dinged it rather lightly for a major offense. When the surveyors moved on to Mission Hill, however, the facility received a major "scolding" as follows:

Dietary order read 1 glass of cranberry juice with breakfast.

Resident requested only 1/2 glass this AM.

No corrective order to document the change from 1 glass to 1/2 glass was written, and yet surveyor found 1/2 glass.

The survey team concluded that documentation must be improved.

Zoë responded in kind. She wrote a clarification order to be placed on all breakfast trays that contained cranberry juice, which read as follows:

"Resident may receive 1/2 to 1 glass of cranberry juice each morning, per daily request of said resident."

After some wrangling back and forth with the state, Mission Hill prevailed. The facility was not cited on the juice issue. Still, a tiny variable in the morning routine, which had been up in the air, now had been nailed down by the state and our able Zoë.

There was a cost. Energy, which could be spent on direct care—and time, which could be spent with the residents—instead were diverted to implement and document such trifles. Such exertions also helped to explain why Zoë was never a popular person on staff.

There is another nuance at work here, too. Eventually, we may begin to believe that the rule to document the amount of juice that may be poured into a glass each morning has some profounder meaning than meets the eye. Conversely, if we disregard one rule, we may begin to disregard others, some of which may be truly important. Conflicts over which rules to obey and which to ignore can begin to undermine the cohesiveness of the care team, at least in cases where a strong friendship is not in place, like the one that I have with Carol Sue.

In my own practice, I have watched even the excellent care team at Mission Hill move away from reliance on individual decision making based on knowledge, experience, and judgment, in favor of rules that anticipate every move. I worry, too, that even at Mission Hill the staff will soon become a unit whose only task is to robotically follow the guidelines and to solve problems in the only way it will know how—by creating more rules.

In the case of long-term care, there is so much that we cannot change for residents—aging, suffering, loss, and death—and there is much that we cannot change for ourselves, that is, for those of us that staff nursing homes. Our needs largely go unmet for meaningful work and for satisfying relationships with our peers and the people we serve. To mask our helplessness, we turn to rules. We disguise the inevitable by making the simple complex. We might try instead to simplify what we can in a complex world.

Common sense should tell us that no expert intervention is required to administer a cough drop, which a child can buy at the local convenience store. Just a decade ago, when so many forms of communication did not exist, neither did the rules that regulated the administration of cough drops. Physicians and nurses are called on more often now—because we can be readily reached—via pager, voice mail, fax, cell phone, e-mail, and land line. Our real value is being diluted as we answer these calls. Our skills are misconstrued and misunderstood, governed as we are by trivia.

There is no evidence that the rise in nursing home rules has had a positive effect on patient care, or that our greater accessibility as caregivers means that we take better care of our elderly and infirm. Mission Hill, it is true, still does a good job, and its normal care team does have a statistically better chance of achieving good outcomes. As we will see elsewhere, however, people living in long-term care facilities consistently lack high-quality care, as caring professionals themselves are degraded by a theory of care. We that work in the field, I fear, are being asked to serve a belief system based on rules that lead self-servingly straight back to themselves, and do not serve the real needs of real people. Will we soon be required to believe in Santa, too?

Four
False Serenity

I cannot say that I always dread going to Serenity Acres, but usually I do. I anticipate the day in the week that I will visit there, not by my calendar, but by my angst when my alarm clock rings in the morning. I used to chalk up my discomfort to midweek blues, but when my schedule changed and I started visiting on a Monday, and then a Friday, the same old feelings did not get chased away. I find it no coincidence that the facility's nickname is "the Acres." It would be too ironic to equate the place with peace.

If Mission Hill offers what I term normal care, Serenity Acres is its opposite. Here the care team is dysfunctional. Staff members tend to bicker and hold conflicting opinions as to how to treat residents and each other. The quality of care they offer is uneven, to say the least. Communication with the residents and their families is inconsistent and often incoherent. Sometimes information is not relayed at all. Everyone takes a turn at being frustrated, angry, and confused.

My own unease is probably best illustrated in terms of certain incidents. I recall, for example, when Maxine Combes, an erstwhile administrator at the Acres, asked me to evaluate a resident the next morning and fill out the form required for a much-needed emergency guardianship.

"I'll get Jamie, the new business manager, to put the form in your box tonight," Maxine assured me.

The next morning I walked into the facility mailroom to look for the document I needed to complete and sign. It was not there. Before I could begin quietly cursing Jamie's incompetence, there she was before me.

"Dr. Silber, did you find the paper Maxine needs you to complete?"

When I told her I had not, she recounted events as though we were two characters in a detective novel.

"I left the papers in your mailbox myself. It was last evening, at about ten o'clock," she said. "Tell me, doctor, was the door locked when you entered this morning?"

"No," I said, slightly taken aback. "It wasn't, but I've never known the mailroom to be locked."

"Well, we've had some problems with the mailboxes," Jamie said. "I'll have another document delivered to you later today."

I could tell that she did not want to elaborate. I could only guess that there was some type of tampering or theft, but why would anyone want to take random pieces of mail in the middle of the night from a nursing home? The mystery will probably never be solved, or at least I do not expect to be informed if it ever is.

Already I was aware of how casually, if not carelessly, the Acres handled mail. A few weeks before, I had spotted a pile of envelopes on the floor behind the nurses' station. When I stooped to get a good look, I could see the pile consisted of unopened mail, postmarked about two weeks earlier. Some of it was junk, but most pieces were bills and personal letters sent to the residents.

"Why is this mail sitting on the floor? Shouldn't it be sorted and delivered?"

I asked several staff members these questions. No one had answers, although everyone seemed nonchalant.

Finally, someone did come over and pick up the mail but only to drop it into a corner of the receptionist's cubicle. There it sat, until one day it was gone. I have no idea whether it was delivered or if it simply disappeared.

Why was I the only person to comment on a pile of mail right under the noses of staff, who sat at the nurses' station all day long? And why, once I asked questions, was the mail simply moved from one state of limbo to another?

Less mysterious is why I serve at Serenity Acres. There are several good reasons. The Acres is close to home, which means that I do not have to commute nearly as far as I usually do. I am the facility medical director and the physician to the overwhelming majority of the residents—nearly one hundred—and generally maintain my monopoly. Unpredictable staffing levels in a chaotic environment scare other doctors away. The few that do venture into the facility do not stay.

I have come to expect randomness instead of routine, as well as transience and absenteeism of the employees, even those in upper management. Still, as I have said, low expectations have not rid me of my apprehension, despite the fact that I am on-site at least once a week and speak to the staff at least three or four times a day. There is always a surprise, a setback, or an aggravation.

As part of my contract as the facility medical director, I provide a physical exam to each new employee, which takes between fifteen and thirty minutes to perform. I have offered this service once a week at the Acres for more than ten years and, by my calculation, performed the exam more than five hundred times. Despite the regularity of these exams, however, I have never succeeded in getting from the facility the three things I need to do the job: a room with a door and two chairs; the appearance at a set time of the two to five employees that will undergo the examination; and a form for each examinee, ready for me to fill out. Instead every week turns out to be a brand new experience. Where are the forms? What room will I use? Where are the people I am supposed to examine?

Appearances Deceive

It may come as a surprise to know that, on the surface, the Acres appears to be the very model of a nursing home—even quite an attractive, upscale one—its lobby graced by pale carpets and a pair of chandeliers. It is just that the surface is wafer thin.

Nestled in a good part of town, the facility attracts older people nearby, who find the proximity to their own homes reassuring. Elderly neighbors are not enough, however, to fill the Acres to capacity, so corporate owners seek supplemental, "alternative" residents for the purpose. Some of these extras include registered sex offenders and aging ex-convicts, whose room and board Medicaid or Medicare can be relied on to pay. Mixed indiscriminately among the rest of the residents, these irregulars do have something—although far from everything—to do with the dysfunction that characterizes facility operations.

Typically, I arrive at the Acres at six-thirty in the morning, a time when the facility door is still locked for the previous night. I bang on the door, but usually no one answers. A few staff members exit the building as they come off the night shift. Intent on the parking lot, they shuffle past me without a glance. I could try and grab hold of the door as they exit, but I do not wish to enter the building without an escort. The chaos of the place breeds a tense atmosphere—too tense for me to suddenly appear out of nowhere. Instead I call into the facility with my cell phone (not too pleasant in the rain). After multiple rings, the phone is answered. Someone is sent to let me in, grudgingly. I start my day in the nursing supervisor's office, where I go through the papers and forms left for me in my mailbox. Here I am taken for granted, as the old hand that I am, and blend in like the proverbial fly on the wall. All around me, talk continues unabated and uncensored.

Because of the change in shifts, the room is filled with nurses and nursing assistants, as well as the night and day nursing supervisors. Much of the conversation consists of bickering over who will work which unit that day. The conversation is punctuated by emergency phone calls, which the night supervisor is making to staffing agencies, as she tries to fill the slots that will otherwise remain empty, because of absenteeism or job vacancy, or because some of the agency employees, already hired, have canceled at the last minute or have simply failed to show up.

As a consequence several units do not have a nurse, and medications and treatments already are due. The nurses who are here will have to pull extra duty to compensate for the loss of unit coverage. Not surprisingly, several nursing assistants say they will complain to Maxine Combes, the administrator. The laundry workers, meanwhile, did not do their job last night. Two out of the five units are without clean clothes; their residents will have to wear hospital gowns today.

By eight, the supervisor's room is nearly empty, with staff on their way to their assigned units. Only the two nursing supervisors remain: Delores Maynard, coming off the night shift, and Patty King, coming on for the day. Delores recaps how awful it is to be short-staffed and how tough it is to deal with the stress. I sympathize but say nothing, not wishing to call attention to myself. Either they have forgotten my presence or feel comfortable enough to ignore me.

"Helluva morning after a helluva night," Patty agrees. "I can't believe I totally forgot to do an IV antibiotic on that young guy in 3B. You know, the one with the infected prosthetic knee joint. I feel horrible, but what a zoo, huh?"

Patty does not actually sound upset, however, and she quickly changes the subject. "Katie got a birthday gift from Maxine, but I didn't. And I've been here way longer."

Delores replies, "Don't you know? Rumor has it, the ladies are lovers. Do you want to do that just to get a $25 gift certificate?"

I am left to wonder when Jeff Howard will get his medication. He could lose his leg if his infection is not treated properly. Diligence and accuracy in treatment are key. Unfortunately, all I can do is prescribe medication, and a patient does not always keep tabs on what is given to him and when. Quietly I get up and leave to make my rounds. I will check on Jeff myself today and see what I can find out.

Still a little low on caffeine, I feel a bit dreamy, when a second thought enters my mind. If Jeff does lose his leg, the facility will have another permanent placement. A bit far-fetched, but who knows? It is not unusual for my alert residents to tell me that they rarely get their medications when a nurse from a temporary staffing agency is on duty. Patty King knocked herself out this morning to meet regulations that call for a body to fill every vacant position. Problem is, the quality of the service rendered is not guaranteed.

Technically, none of these matters are my business. I am here to visit patients in the facility, which I do with little difficulty. It is only when I am on my way out the door of the Acres that the housekeeper runs out to stop me.

"Didn't the nurse tell you about the new resident upstairs—the one who is coughing a lot and turning blue?"

"No," I replied. I had been upstairs for thirty minutes, and no one had told me about anyone new, sick or otherwise.

At the Acres, dealing with acute, preventable crises is the order of the day, largely because no foresight or planning goes into facility management and operations. Now here I was, intercepted at the last minute to put out one more fire. I walked back into the building to see the ill resident.

On my return upstairs, I noticed a nurse, busy writing up one of the morning's incidents in a chart. Quite possibly, her version would not reflect what happened so much as it would conform to the care plan of the resident involved. At the same moment, a sick resident was so badly in need of medical attention that I had to be summoned from the parking lot.

What if I followed the nurse's suit? I could jot something into the sick man's chart, which sounded plausible as to his condition and care, but not go in and see him. Or I could go in and do a thorough assessment of the man but enter nothing at all into his chart. Either way, would it make a difference in his nursing care?

I had to wonder, given it was the Acres. The care plan itself would not be read like the Bible, the way it would be at Mission Hill. Actual care would be a matter of luck and of whim, depending on who was on duty and when.

As to which inaction on my part would be punished more severely, were it ever to surface, the absence of a paper trail would surely be the greater transgression, if for no other reason than because several staff would have witnessed the physical exam and expected to find it written up in the man's chart. Had I not troubled myself to see the sick man in the first place, however, it is not clear that I would have paid any price at all.

Easy Come, Easy Go

Transience is endemic at the Acres. If I become attached to a staff member, or a resident, before I know it, he or she will be asked to leave, or just vanish on his or her own.

In the fifteen years that I have practiced there, I have seen come and go thirteen administrators, seven directors of nursing, and an exponentially large number of nurses, certified nurse assistants, and other staff.

Competence is another matter. In fact, it is rare enough to celebrate—and to mourn when it is gone again. Last January the facility somehow managed to hire Adele Sandler, a highly capable director of nursing. She was knowledgeable, pleasant, and caring. She was experienced in administrative issues such as nursing home regulations and staffing disputes. She worked long hours and was quite dedicated. I dared not get my hopes up that she would stay.

About nine months later, Adele disappeared. Told that she resigned, I was a bit surprised as to how abruptly she had done so. I had not had the chance to say goodbye. Gradually, the full story unfolded. It seemed Adele's dad had taken ill and passed away quickly. State inspectors were in the facility on the day of his funeral. Adele was permitted to take leave for a few hours but was not given the full day off. What kind of a "care" team was this? Many of the more alert residents raised the same question with regard to themselves. The answer was a sad lament: Their caregiver "family" was a joke, if not a farce.

Careless Caregivers

If such a judgment sounds harsh, it is a verdict that reflects the deep disappointment of the frail and the lonely. And, of course, it should come as no surprise. A chaotic, dysfunctional facility is unlikely to attract and to keep competent, industrious staff. Yet to provide a fully rounded sense of how people live and work in American long-term care facilities today, it is best to introduce some of the many individual staff members that have come and gone from the Acres and let their actions speak for themselves.

Amy Gaston provides a good example of someone whose behavior leads me to place her within my "Gallery of Rogues," a designation that unfortunately is not a rarity. Amy was a young licensed practical nurse when I first met her at Mission Hill. In fairness, I must say that she is one of the few staff members with whom I have never had a good relationship. There was something that bothered me from the outset, and it took me quite a while to pinpoint. As it turned out, the answer was simple. She did not do her job well and had trouble showing up to work. As would become clear, she tried to compensate for her shortcomings by lying about other people, and kissing up to higher level staff.

Mission Hill warned Amy several times about her job security, but these warnings did not stop her from being either tardy or absent on a regular basis. She was always less than friendly to me, which did not bother me much. Two incidents, however, did bother me a good deal. The first involved a prescription for a narcotic, which I gave her to have filled for a resident. A week later, she said that she never received my order. I supposed that I could have been mistaken and did not actually hand the slip of paper to her after all, but I did not think so.

The second incident began when I stopped at the nurses' station one day as I was making my rounds. I had a short chat with Amy, who spoke of nothing out of the ordinary. A few hours later, I received a call from the irate son of one of my patients.

"Why didn't you visit my mother today?"

"I saw her two days ago, and she was doing fine," I said, taken aback. "Is something wrong?"

"I told the nurse on duty to be sure and have you check out Mom's left eye when you made your rounds. She seems to have an infection or at least her eye is red and irritated."

"I had no idea."

"Of course you didn't," the man snapped. "The nurse said to forget it. You were too busy to see Mom. If you're that damn busy, I want to switch physicians."

I managed to assuage the woman's son. I also referred the incident to the director of nursing and to the administrator.

Mission Hill fired Amy, largely for absenteeism. The final straw had been my complaint.

For several years thereafter, she worked through an agency that provided temporary staffing at numerous facilities, including the Acres. I conveyed my bad experiences with Amy to the administrator, who listened intently but did not act on my recommendations to avoid using Amy.

On the contrary, Amy began to work as a temporary floor nurse at the Acres. It was not as if she changed her ways. She was tardy still, and absent often. At the Acres, of course, these shortcomings were not out of the ordinary but were tolerated as something close to the norm.

Amy became friendly with Delores Maynard, the day nursing supervisor, who also worked as a temp through the same staffing agency. Delores often called in sick, or else came to work drunk, not that she stayed long. She and Amy carpooled together and developed a habit of punching in and then driving off somewhere during their shift. Such shenanigans went on for a few months until Amy disappeared, the reasons for her departure a mystery. Later I learned that she had stolen money from a resident. I certainly was not surprised.

Six months later, Amy was back on the scene, this time as a permanent hire on the Acres' staff. Within a few weeks, she received a promotion to replace her supervisor, who had upped and quit one day. Now she was the facility treatment nurse and received a week's orientation and training for this advanced position. What happened to the old treatment nurse?

Despair Follows Dysfunction

Like Amy, Mary Holcomb had started at the Acres as a floor nurse. Any resemblance between the two ended there, however. Mary was a good worker but a quiet person. It took time for her to make friends. Few people at the Acres knew that she suffered from a severe manic-depressive illness, which she controlled with numerous medications.

Over time, Mary grew more relaxed and outgoing, even as she continued to excel at doling out medications and treatments on time, and in keeping her notes up-to-date and accurate. Eventually, Maxine Combes saw fit to oversee a "trading places" scheme, in which Mary was promoted to treatment nurse, whereas her predecessor, Heidi Schrum, was demoted to take her place as a floor nurse.

The job swap was fair enough. Heidi had been a floor nurse at the Acres for about ten years. For about five of those years, she had served as a treatment nurse, and, by all accounts, had provided substandard care. Another rogue in my gallery, her documentation was poor, and her work was sloppy. Rumor had it that the state survey team planned to concentrate on treatment documentation during its annual inspection. Heidi had to go.

Mary thrived in her new position. Treatments were done properly and on time; wounds healed. Documentation was updated and immediately placed in the charts. A month after Mary started her new job, the facility underwent a mock survey to prepare for the upcoming state inspection. Results showed that everything was in order, and outcomes were good—in fact, they were better than the state average. Mary was honored as Top Employee of the Month, which came with a coveted perk, namely a special parking spot in front of the facility entrance. Administrative staff took her out to lunch.

A few weeks later, the state inspection team arrived. Astonishingly, they found crucial information missing in many instances. Yet the very items missing had been in their rightful places as recently as the mock survey. What had happened? No one had an answer, except the inspectors, who cited the facility for many violations, and left orders for a whole raft of corrections.

Mary stopped coming to work. Given her reliability, her absence gave rise to concern. After a few days passed with no sign or word from her, one of her closest colleagues paid a visit to Mary's home. There he found her, dead of an overdose.

Despite the Acres' delinquent mail system, it was not long before several staff members found farewell notes from Mary in their facility mailboxes. Her thoughts were not pleasant. What she had written were the words of a disturbed woman, who had toiled in a troubled environment that was not always friendly.

Morale at the Acres could hardly have been lower. The facility was operating under a double burden. Its residents were in need of a treatment nurse, and the state was holding it accountable for a mountain of deficient documentation.

Beautiful Lies

After her demotion to floor nurse, Heidi Schrum had gone to work on the Peach Unit, the facility's dementia and behavioral ward, which I visited once a week. No matter when I arrived or how long I stayed—a half-hour, an hour, or more—Heidi was never to be seen. Whenever I asked after her, she was said to be away on break. Peach was a difficult unit. The residents wandered and were prone to sudden outbursts. To complain about poor care was well beyond most of them. Deeply disoriented, most of them truly were at the staff's mercy. If the residents were not bathed or fed, someone would have sounded an alarm, but if a resident did not get his blood pressure pill, few would have been the wiser. As long as his chart said that he had received the pill, all was well. The fact that he received proper care was a matter of record—what was documented. What should be true was easy enough to put on paper. A floor nurse could document that a pill had been administered, and could write up a perfect blood pressure. The truth could be manufactured.

The possibility that Heidi was cooking the books, so to speak, did cross my mind. Oddities made me wonder. One resident, for instance, showed a high blood level for a drug that she was not supposed to be taking—lab error, perhaps. Yet the hard fact remained. Behaviors on the Peach Unit looked much better on paper when Heidi was on duty, despite the fact that much of the time she was not even there.

Despite Heidi's poor skills and her lack of a work ethic, the administrator and the director of nursing always seemed pleased with her, no doubt because of the beauty of her documentation. After Mary's disappearance, they offered Heidi the job of treatment nurse, seeming to forget that she had been demoted from that very position not long ago. Heidi declined—because she was so happy on the Peach Unit—or so she said. In truth, when actual nursing needed to be done, Heidi was of little use. It took more than words to care for a wound, and Heidi knew it. In actuality, poor work and false recordkeeping went hand in hand here, despite her superiors' failure to notice. They trusted—but did not verify—Heidi's "flawless" documentation.

It was Amy Gaston, then, who got the job. Months went by during which she came to work sporadically, provided minimal treatment, and filed no documentation. Only when state inspectors were due in for their reinspection did matters come to a head. Crisis mode was the Acres' modus operandi, after all. At the eleventh hour, Amy was given the sack in a desperate attempt to fill in the blanks that had caused the earlier inspection disaster.

Again Heidi was offered the treatment nurse's job, this time with a substantial raise, and this time she accepted. Shortly thereafter, the documents that had disappeared on Mary Holcomb's watch began to resurface: in residents' rooms, under stacks of old books, and in mislabeled charts. Heidi was considered a miracle worker: In the nick of time, she had brought back from oblivion the very information needed to satisfy the state inspectors. Although she basked in considerable glory, Heidi did leave the Acres eventually and went on to make far more money as a highly paid agency nurse. As such, she worked in nearly every nursing home in the city.

Apathy and Indifference

Not only does the facility depend heavily on agencies for nurses and aides but also for supervisors, who work a day or two at a time for a hefty fee. The Acres suffers, because supervisory tasks are carried out by people who lack familiarity with the facility and any commitment to it.

During Christmas week a few years ago, for example, agency supervisors took the lead, when most permanent staff members were absent. I was shocked to find a few of the residents themselves acting as supervisors as they guided temporary staff to the medicine cabinet and the linen room. One resident actually played receptionist, and answered the unit's telephone, although not very successfully. Could such a motley crew call itself a care team? It could and did at the Acres.

Occasionally, I welcome agency staff as a much-needed reprieve from their permanent counterparts, whose shortcomings are only too well known and long endured. After just a few days, however, it is the return of the subpar regulars that comes as a relief. Temporary workers can be the most irresponsible of them all, particularly in a facility with a care team as dysfunctional as the one at the Acres. An agency nurse that goes AWOL may be placed on the "do not rehire" list. A few weeks later, however, she will be back on the job.

Yet many competent caregivers do work for agencies. I recall a very able nurse, who took the time to explain to several of us why she was leaving the Acres to work for an agency. The downside would be the challenge of working at a new place most days, and no guarantee of a full schedule. The attraction, she claimed, was that the agency would provide more stability than the Acres, given how quickly changes had occurred there and what little control she had had over her schedule or floor assignments. As for health benefits, she would be paid enough to afford her own. Skeptical at first, we soon began to see her point.

Mañana, Mañana, Maxine

Instability and chaos lead to transience and absenteeism. Transience and absenteeism lead to instability and chaos. The circle is vicious, and the proverbial chicken-and-egg question has no answer. As already mentioned, I have witnessed thirteen administrators come and go from the Acres. Maxine Combes herself filled the role on four separate occasions. Her total time on the job amounted to about two years. The first three times, she quit on her own accord, largely in recognition of her own inadequacies.

In her forties, Maxine was close to my own age and very kind. Staff and residents liked her, and she showed an unusual level of commitment to the Acres; her own sister was a resident at one point. She always was willing to listen to complaints and issues with concern and sympathy. The problem was that Maxine did little planning and even less follow-up on any issue or concern that arose. Day-to-day operational decisions were forever deferred; problems were left to accumulate, and conflicts to fester, unresolved. The staff worked in a state of perpetual anxiety until a crisis arose and brought with it some dysfunctional form of relief.

During her fourth attempt to run the facility, Maxine suddenly found herself terminated. Over night, she cleared out her desk, and her family photos vanished off the wall. Corporate told us that she had resigned. However, she did not say goodbye to anyone, the way she had in the past, which was not like her. Maxine had always been gracious and considerate. Although she could rarely make a decision, she was a firm believer in sharing every bit of information with staff.

For a few months, the facility hovered under a cloud of disquiet, as we wondered what had led Maxine to leave in such an uncharacteristic way. Yet to ask for an explanation was out of the question, the new administrator clearly implied.

The Acres has also seen many directors of nursing come and go, with an average stay of about four months. Most are not even a blip on my radar. Once, in fact, I found myself saying goodbye to someone I had not even realized had been serving as a director of nursing, such a very short time had it been. Most directors have left voluntarily, but a few have been asked to leave. Elaine Potter fell into the latter category.

Her first words to me were, "We're going to find a real doctor to serve here."

Like many a bully, she wrote up the good nurses but somehow left the substandard ones alone.

She certainly made her mark. Aggressive and intrusive, her most lasting legacy was an exodus of employees—numerous aides, three long-term nurses, and even the custodian of twenty-five years' standing—all of whom quit during her tenure. Thus she managed to profoundly scar the facility, which was quite a feat, given its impervious nature.

At one point, I entertained the thought of leaving myself. Yet I had a hunch that Elaine would not last long, and right I was. Within three months, the administrator at the time let her go. (Had Maxine been in charge, I would not have been optimistic, given her indecisiveness.)

Physicians in Flight

Transience at the Acres extends to attending physicians. During the last fifteen years, I have been the only doctor to remain for long. My Gallery of Rogues includes a few of these doctors, who have come and gone. For better and for worse, it is thanks to them that my patient load at the Acres is so very large.

Occasionally a young doctor like Abner Collins will arrive to build his practice. If Abner lasted a little longer than most, perhaps it was because he arrived with the attitude that he alone could solve all of the Acres' considerable problems. Eventually, even he became frustrated and quit without leaving so much as a phone number or other way to contact him. I was obliged to step in and take his residents under my care.

I thought that we had heard the end of Dr. Collins, but I was wrong. He went on to work at a local hospital, to which residents from the Acres were admitted from time to time, and he badmouthed the facility whenever the opportunity presented itself, as we shall later see.

Inez Perez was another doctor whose tenure at the Acres was decidedly brief, even though she arrived with considerable experience gained in convalescent homes. For a month or so, she made her rounds uneventfully. Then she began to complain—first about a floor nurse, and then about Margo Kennedy, the day supervisor at the time. Dr. Perez did not seem to realize that, no matter how badly staff were performing, the administrative office did not want to hear about it; frankly any complaint was frowned on. One thing led to another, until Dr. Perez called corporate headquarters to offer her resignation. I was sorry to see her go.

The upshot was that I was left to care for practically every patient in the facility, which was not a good thing, especially as the number of residents was growing. They deserved a choice in physicians, and I welcomed some relief and mutual support from a colleague. The Acres recruited Karl Peterson, who agreed to take on a limited caseload. Delighted, I left for vacation under the impression that he would arrive during my absence and take on ten new residents as his patients.

Two weeks later I returned to find that not only had Dr. Peterson seen all of the new admissions but had also taken on about twenty of my regular patients, who had transferred their care to him. Distraught, I went to see Maxine.

"Were the residents not satisfied with my care?" I asked.

"Well, of course they're satisfied. There must be some misunderstanding," she said, though she had no inkling of what it might be.

It was left to a floor nurse to clue me in: "They were told that you no longer wanted to take care of them," she told me.

"Who told them?" I demanded but never did get an answer.

As often was the case at the Acres, the problem faded as mysteriously as it arose. Before long, my former patients had returned to me.

Common Sense, a Saving Grace

Patty King had served as the day supervisor of nursing for several years, which made her an old-timer at the Acres. She shared her responsibilities with Margo Kennedy, and each worked alternately, each pulling a twelve-hour shift. Their styles were as opposing as their schedules. At first I had mixed feelings about them both. I preferred Patty when Margo was working and Margo when Patty was.

In her forties, Patty was close to my age but appeared twenty years older; she had packed a lot of hardship into the same years. Like so many of the staff, she had a large family, financial problems, and struggled with alcohol. Most weeks, she made it to work four out of the five days that she was on duty. Three of those four days, she either would leave early or come in late. Although I did not condone her absenteeism, I could sympathize.

Patty was not a great worker, but she was not the worst. True, she usually did a sloppy job and wrote orders late, if at all. The pleasant surprise was that, just as often, she showed stellar judgment. She would scan the list of care team recommendations and pick out the ones that counted as far as patient care was concerned. Patty happened to have common sense, a much underrated trait in my experience. We can learn medical science, but practical application is an art. Patty did not call me often, but when she did, she had good reason.

Patty's father passed away rather suddenly of a quickly progressing cancer. Her mother, who was in her early sixties, became very ill thereafter. After an extensive hospitalization, she came to convalesce at the Acres. I was a bit surprised, given that Patty openly criticized the care at the facility as poor.

"I want her near me," was her explanation. "And I want her near you, too."

Thus Patty's mom became my patient. I became very close to Muriel, and paid her special attention, not because she was Patty's mom, but because I grew to love her. She adored dragonflies, as did my youngest daughter. The two became friends by proxy, although they never met. Eventually Muriel spread her wings and flew into another world. Overstressed by work and now in anguish, Patty quit her job. I did not know which woman I would miss more.

Computing Conscientiously

Patty's counterpart also had been on staff a long time, at least by the standards of the Acres. Unlike Patty, Margo lacked commonsense and independent judgment. A conversation with her never was simple or quick. If I plotted a graph of the number of calls that I received per day, I would know which days she had been on duty. Sometimes she called ten or fifteen times in a twelve-hour shift. Whenever I received a page with three voice mails, I knew who my caller had to be.

Margo's messages were so verbose that often she would need to call back three times to say what was on her mind. To listen to a question took far longer than it did to answer. Sometimes when I returned her call, she would still be in the process of leaving me the message to which I was responding. To top it off, sometimes she could not remember why she had called me to begin with, even when I responded immediately. If she did remember, she would repeat her voice-mail message in its entirety.

To protect my sanity, I learned to be blunt with Margo. However, my brusqueness did not make her any less prolix. I took a deep breath every time I called her back. I would try my best not to lose my cool, but on occasion I would.

Perhaps the most peculiar aspect of her interrogations was her demand for canned responses—ones that would match perfectly a normative list she had found somewhere.

To satisfy her I needed to say such things as, "No new orders," or "Get a chest x-ray." Statements such as, "Let's think about it for a day and see what happens," or "Let's do nothing now," were completely unacceptable.

To most people, "No new orders," and "Let's do nothing now," would be equivalent propositions. Margo, however, was unable to make the translation. Like a computer program, she was unable to process unless she received an answer in just the right format.

Similarly, Margo had no way to prioritize. She treated all problems as equally urgent. The alcohol content in a gift box of bourbon balls was as of much concern as a dying resident. She repeated each problem ad nauseam until she received her acceptable answer.

She was someone to avoid, if I could, and to dispatch as quickly as possible when we needed to communicate. Then one morning I overhead one nurse say to another, "Margo Kennedy says she and Dr. Silber are best friends. Isn't that a riot?"

The two women guffawed.

So Margo was a laughingstock. I should not have been surprised.

It appeared that I was among the few willing to take her seriously. There and then I stopped being exasperated. Never again would I take a deep breath before I answered her calls. I was not really her friend, but I could offer her support. Then it occurred to me why: She deserved my respect. She had earned an A+ for conscientiousness aboard our drifting ship.

Five
Corporate Care Mongering

Although Serenity Acres feels adrift, it is in fact part of a conglomerate—Golden Springs Healthcare Systems—which includes some thirty facilities across several states. Corporate owner John Huntington buys old, poorly run nursing homes and turns them around. Within a few months of acquisition, beds are filled and so are coffers. Miraculously these facilities fare quite well during state inspection surveys, despite characteristically substandard care and poor staffing of the kind to be found at the Acres. John is a somewhat infamous character in the long-term care community, and he is rumored to have political ties. He is respected for his success but distrusted for his possibly less-than-caring business transactions that keep the bottom line in the crosshairs.

John does make it a point to treat very well the physicians that work for him. As a bit player in his empire, I am paid a good stipend as the Acres' medical director—and always on time—a rarity in this business. If I express a concern, it is usually taken into consideration. If nothing comes of it, at least I am recognized and heard. Most corporate offices do not extend this courtesy, nor do they make me feel appreciated. Golden Springs always sends a nice holiday gift and a gift for Doctor's Day. Its managers go the extra mile to accommodate their special guests. When I was invited to give a dinner talk one evening in the corporate dining room, another doctor requested a special drink. The bar did not have on hand all of the necessary ingredients. The marketing director jumped up from the table and went straight out to purchase them. He returned with fresh cream and coffee liqueur and fixed the drink himself.

Image Boosts and Image Boots

Most corporate involvement with individual facilities has to do with efforts to boost their image. Such enhancements are presented with much fuss and bother but then are quickly forgotten as a passing fancy, much like the White Russian cocktail, which the marketing director concocted to impress my colleague. On several occasions, Serenity Acres underwent a name change: Serenity Mount became the Manor at Serenity and then the Manor at Nature's Edge. All four nursing stations were rechristened in honor of beautiful flowers and sweet fruits, such as the peach, which denotes the Acres' dementia and behavioral unit.

Sometimes, however, the search for a better image can be traumatic for the residents. When the Acres was renamed the Manor at Serenity, for instance, a major shift occurred in the population. Residents known to be troublesome or particularly unattractive were made to move into other nearby corporate facilities, whereas better-behaved, better-looking people arrived from elsewhere to create what corporate managers called an "upgrade in atmosphere." In a similar if less drastic scheme several years later, so-called problem residents whose rooms happened to be on the first floor and near the main entrance one day found themselves relocated into the back corridors. The relocation had come in tandem with another change in the facility name, prompting one resident to comment: "Let's change the name one more time, and maybe people will forget that this is a shitty place."

All a Façade

Public image has always been the Acres' strong suit. The dysfunction of its operations is well hidden. A visitor would have to be exceptionally astute, or else camp out for a good, long time to get an inkling of the true state of affairs.

Nearly always filled to capacity, the credit for its full house goes largely to the superb marketing team that Golden Springs employs to impress prospective residents. One of these employees works at the Acres and scouts residents within a 100-mile radius. Two additional corporate marketers look for prospects nationwide and often jet around the country to do so.

It would be difficult to accuse the corporation of discrimination or exclusivity. Prisoners on parole and the homeless have found their way to Golden Springs' facilities, as have some desperate survivors of Hurricane Katrina.

The Acres keep its secrets, largely because it maintains a very good documentation system. Care plans are adhered to on paper regardless of what actually is done. It helps, too, that there is no institutional memory, as so few staff members stay long enough to know what is going on, and a large percentage of the workforce is made up of temporary workers, who are on-site only a few days at a time. The few people that have been on staff for a long time appear to have lost track of the facility's irregularities and no longer recognize the problems all around them. A very few, such as Margo Kennedy, are blinded by devotion.

In short, Golden Springs markets a substandard product. It is packaged well and has an attractive wrapper—the care plan—but is defective where it counts, namely, in the quality of its nursing. Yet, the marketing team has no problem selling the Acres. It is a product that continues to fly off the shelf.

A Mockery of Standards

The wizardry of marketing will only take a facility so far, however. A nursing home's capability to undergo the state survey process and survive, if not excel, remains critical to its viability. Mock surveys have become the way to prepare in advance for a state inspection team. A corporation either conducts the practice tests internally, or an outside agency is called in to perform them for a fee. Sometimes both methods are used. In large conglomerates, such as the one that the Acres belongs to, a team of mock surveyors is employed to go from facility to facility and perform mock surveys. Such rituals seem to have taken on a life of their own. They tend to distract staff from what should be our real focus, namely providing excellent care to our residents.

Facilities are told when to expect the corporation's mock team, unlike the real team whose arrival is meant to come as a surprise. The last time a mock team arrived at the Acres, it began its three-day stint on the Plum Unit. Staff members were well-dressed and on their best behavior, as were the residents, and the facility's typical skeleton crew had been fleshed out with supposedly qualified agency workers.

If all went well and the facility passed the survey, everyone would celebrate with a catered feast.

If the facility did not pass, however, upper management could expect to be let go and replaced with a new team, or an interim team—never a good outcome for lower level staff.

I had little involvement in the mock survey process myself, other than to observe and record the proceedings. Here are a few of my favorite exchanges, which include the responses that residents were urged to give—in addition to the genuine but ignored answers of those participants too irrepressible or disgruntled to stick to their scripts.

Mock Survey Team Member: "Mrs. Getty, do you feel that the care you receive is good here?"

Scripted Answer: "Yes, I'd recommend it to my friends. I'm happy that my family sent me here."

Real Answer: "No, but I'm afraid to complain. I have nowhere to go. My family doesn't want me. I'm too much of a problem for a good nursing home to take me."

Mock Survey Team Member: "Samantha, do you feel that you can count on the support of the director of nursing, if you are short-staffed?"

Scripted Answer: "Yes, she's always here to help and pass medications and to do treatments if needed."

Real Answer: "I don't really know or care. I just started last week, and it's so horrible here, I may just walk out today." (This nurse did leave after lunch shortly after the mock survey and did not return.)

Mock Survey Team Member: "Peggy, could you explain why there are ten extra antibiotic pills in your medication cart?"

Scripted Answer: "The physician ordered the pill discontinued. I need to notify the pharmacy of that fact."

Real Answer: "I forgot to give them to the patients."

On and on it went. The mock survey continued with a series of questions and responses over three days. The team recorded each of the scripted answers, reviewed each resident's actual care plan, and then produced a report.

Despite the enormous effort, the fact remained: Serenity Acres did not provide good care. Were they asked to be honest, most people that worked there and most people that conducted its surveys, mock or real, would attest to this simple, sad fact.

By contrast, two other facilities that I serve have both received a dismal rating by a national public watchdog organization. The scores are based largely on artificial factors, most of them self-reported. In reality, the care at these facilities is excellent. On paper, however, the Acres looks like the better bet.

Freedom Rings

Luckily, most residents do not really need excellent care to survive, as Carol Sue implied about her mother. They can get by with considerably less.

God help those that cannot.

Jeff Howard was one of them. Dependent on IV antibiotics, he could have lost his leg while one nurse kvetched about not getting a birthday gift from the administrator and the other gossiped about a rumored lesbian romance. At the Acres, residents can count on their medications only when the core staff is on duty, and only then if they are not too preoccupied with their own personal dramas. Yet, by and large, the resident population is quite content. Even people that complain about not getting their medication on time tell me that they are satisfied and treated well.

Perhaps their satisfaction arises from the added personal freedom that chaos and dysfunction afford. It is true that residents at the Acres enjoy fewer restrictions than they would at a better-run facility. Again, consider Jeff Howard. He is what is known in the industry as a "frequent flyer": He moves in and out of long-term care, depending on his health. When he needed another stay in a nursing home and the Acres was full, he asked to be transferred there as soon as possible. Why would he do that? Fiftyish, he would be allowed to share a room with his twenty-year-old girlfriend (also a resident).

Illicit activities like smoking marijuana on the grounds or slipping out for the day against insurance policy are not officially sanctioned at the Acres. They simply go unnoticed or else are shrugged off. Over-the-counter cough drops may be popped at bedside by anyone who wants, unofficially, of course. I guess there is one thing more important than getting your medication on time—autonomy.

A Doctored Diagnosis

Two months after the mock survey, the state came in for its yearly visit. One chart in particular received special scrutiny. It belonged to a patient with many problems, both personal and health-related. Why did her chart receive so much attention?

First, her case involved five major issues, which the state had decided to target that year: weight loss, chronic pain, wounds, poly-pharmaceutical usage, and behavioral problems. Second, the patient, when interviewed, was very angry about her care and was able to give a good story to go along with it.

In her mid-sixties, Nancy Arbenz had been a resident at the Acres for about five years. She had multiple medical and psychiatric issues and, by her own admission, had been "sort of a problem" all of her life. She had three daughters. Two were banned from the facility because of disruptive and inappropriate behavior on numerous occasions. The police were called in on suspicion that the two women were stealing their mother's pain medications and taking them home for themselves. The third and relatively responsible daughter had several serious health problems of her own. Chances were, she would end up in a long-term care facility herself in time. As Carol Sue would say, the apple did not fall far from the tree.

There had never been a time when Mrs. Arbenz and her family did not complain bitterly about the facility and her care. Yet she had nowhere else to go. No other facility would take her and tolerate her disruptive behavior.

Her most pressing problem was pain, she said, which was a puzzle. Nancy, all ninety pounds of her, was on enough pain medications to control the agony of an elephant with an amputated leg. No one could stop the pain. Over the course of thirty years, she had visited clinics, psychiatrists, orthopedists, and neurologists, to no avail.

Although mysterious, the pain had to be documented and continued attempts made to control it. Otherwise, the facility would get a bad rating and perhaps be fined.

The second issue of concern was Nancy's weight loss. Mrs. Arbenz had never been a big eater. Her current circumstances did not improve her appetite. The Acres was not known for fine dining, and Nancy's opiate-induced daze and her difficult relationship with her family were major distractions. Slowly but surely she dwindled over her five-year stay at the Acres. Again, a bad rating or a fine would be in order, unless a plan were in place to reverse the process.

And then there were the falls. Mrs. Arbenz fell and fell and fell. She fell when she was "stoned" on her pain medications. She fell when her family did not visit, and she fell when they did. She fell when she needed to and wanted to. She even fell right in front of the survey team, with fifteen people keeping an eye on her. The saving grace was that she never broke a bone. A bad rating might result, depending on how the state assessed the effort to address the problem, but there would be no significant fine: She had never sustained a serious injury.

Next were the wounds. Nancy had one from an old colostomy, which she insisted on tending to herself. She would not let anyone look at it or care for it. Although she could not be forced to have the wound treated, the survey team did use its authority to force her to have it looked at. The site did not look good: it was macerated, red, and inflamed. What was to be done? Was the facility responsible when the resident refused treatment?

The high number of drugs she used was another serious concern. In her search for pain relief, Nancy had visited at least thirty specialists and subspecialists over the years. She came away dissatisfied unless she received a prescription—or two or three. Nancy was on forty-four medications, and she wanted more. What were we going to do about that?

Last, but not least, were the behavioral issues. She ranted and raved, cried in pain, threatened suicide, and said everyone hated her. For the record, she hated everyone in return. In this case, the problems were thoroughly documented, and interventions were in place. All was well, as far as the state inspectors were concerned.

The facility's corporate gurus were called in to review the chart. A lot was on the line. Given the length of her medical history and the size of her chart—and Mrs. Arbenz did have a very large chart—hope lay in what might be found in the several volumes of documentation. Eventually, there it was. Buried deep in the pages lay a diagnosis of cholagniocarcinoma, a very rare form of cancer, which would justify and account for chronic pain, weight loss, falls, wounds, polypharmacuetical use, and behavioral issues. Voila. The problem was solved. Mrs. Arbenz was made hospice and had a faultless care plan for all of her problems. The survey team backed off and began to examine another chart, that of Betsy Warner, former resident of Mission Hill.

There was a postscript to the case of Mrs. Arbenz. After she passed away some years later, her relatively responsible daughter filed a lawsuit against the facility for neglect and poor care. Once again, corporate sat down and read her chart.

Cholangiocarcimoma was found to be a typo. The typo appeared not once but in a series. On Mrs. Arbenz' initial admission to the facility, the nurse had noted a history of cholecystitis—gallstones in layman's terms. In fact, Nancy had hers removed at one point. It was on her return to the Acres that the admissions nurse entered the mistake into her chart. Mrs. Arbenz' cholecystitis became cholecystoma. During a chart audit, the mistake got compounded. Cholecystoma became cholangioma. Later still, cholangioma became cholangiocarcinoma—gallbladder cancer in layman's terms.

Mrs. Arbenz's benign condition had metastasized into a rare and quickly fatal form of cancer. Through a series of mistakes, the facility had been blessed with an apparent answer to all of its problems, until now.

Now it became clear that Mrs. Arbenz had not died from a rare form of cancer, after all. The facility no longer had a way to explain her chronic pain, weight loss, falls, wounds, polypharmaceutical use, and behavioral issues. Needless to say, the chart was doctored and the typo made consistent throughout. The Acres had to battle charges of neglect, and could hardly afford to admit to such an error. Nancy's true cause of death would have to remain a mystery.

As must be quite clear by now, what actually happens is not necessarily what gets documented and reported. Likewise, the correlation between actual care and reported care may vary considerably.

Poor care is supposed to result in a poor survey, and good care in a positive one. The reality may be vastly different.

At the same time, outcomes for residents are sometimes quite similar—regardless of whether the care team is competent or not. How can that be? Perhaps patients are resilient in the same way as children that grow up in a dysfunctional household and often perform as well as those in a highly functional one. Evolution has bestowed on us the gift of a wide and forgiving margin of error.

As for rules, they can give us a false sense of assurance that we know what we are doing and that we have a good reason for what we do. Neither assumption is necessarily so. Rules can have little to do with the facts on the ground, the reality of a situation, or the needs at stake. They do not necessarily protect people and prevent mistakes. As we have seen, they can be arbitrary and absurd. They may simply be a means to an end, such as winning a game. Yet these rules can loom large, to the extent that they shape games that themselves have taken on monumental importance.

Rules of the Game

Soccer is an example. Undoubtedly the sport is a healthy outlet, so much so that it appears the game has almost become a requirement among school-aged children. If I appear to exaggerate, consider Adele Sandler, the stellar director of nursing at Serenity Acres the very short period that she was there. One morning I found her crying in her office. The problem? She did not have time to transport her kindergartener to soccer because she worked past seven. She had to hire a nanny, which she could not afford, to drive her child to the many practices and then to the games. I asked her if she really needed to make such a financial sacrifice.

She stopped crying and looked up at me in surprise: "What? You don't believe in soccer?"

Taken aback, I realized that, for Adele and many other parents, soccer was more than a game. It was a code of conduct that came with a sort of creed whose "truth" had to be believed.

Sports provide us with expressive outlets, not all of which are necessarily healthy. Our family turned up at a favorite restaurant one evening to find a local television crew busy recording live interviews with members of the Tampa Bay Buccaneers. Right away we noticed that most patrons were wearing team togs and waving team flags and other paraphernalia. Later we learned that these diners were vying to be named "fan of the week."

As we took in the unexpected scene, our son, Jared, stood there at the threshold, emblazoned with the Miami Dolphins' name and logos across his arms and chest. After a moment, he took his beloved jacket off and folded it over his arm, inside out.

How extreme, I thought, even for a shy person like Jared. And yet we were all uncomfortable. I stood there and realized: We were not afraid of this crowd because we were Jewish. We were afraid because we were not big fans of the Tampa Bay Buccaneers.

Have we Americans redirected our deep-seated intolerance? No longer is it socially acceptable to call someone a "kike" or a "dago," but we can express our hatred for fans of rival sports teams, even though the players pledge their allegiance according to their latest contract agreement. Today's Dolphin may be tomorrow's Buccaneer.

Of course it is fine that sports figures inspire us to strive for personal greatness. Celebrity role models can have a positive influence on our lives. Increasingly, however, we tend to mistake the feats and accomplishments of our heroes as our own. Perhaps this blurring is a consequence of commercialism. I doubt that everyone that wears a Harvard or a Yale t-shirt has actually studied at one of those esteemed Ivy League institutions, or even knows someone that has.

Martin's Feather

One of my former patients used to try and help me sort through the contradictions and deceptions, which we all encounter when we live and work in long-term care. Martin Scanlon loved to philosophize and used to tell me something interesting every time I saw him. During one of our last conversations, I mentioned that I had just come from my rounds at Sweet Penny Tree, a nursing home where Mr. Scanlon had once resided. He asked me about several of his favorite staff members there, and I gave him what gossip I could. Then I told him what was really going on over there. It was a chance to vent. Given his weakened state, I did not think he would comprehend everything I told him, namely that the corporation that owned Sweet

Penny Tree had just acquired a local hospice. Sweet Penny management had instructed the director of nursing to start to evaluate residents to see who might be appropriate for related services.

It was not long before I got a call from a man whose mother was in my care. He told me that the nursing home recommended that Mom enter hospice. "Is she dying, doctor? Should I hop a plane and come see her?"

Although she was quite ill, the woman's status had remained stable for many years. What was I to tell him? That we needed to make money and that, statistically speaking, his mother was likely to die soon? Or should I have said that the facility hoped to designate as hospice all residents without good payment plans? After all, was not life itself a terminal illness?

Diplomatically, I opted to say that we were trying to give his mother the best care available, and it was through hospice that we could do so.

Mr. Scanlon heard and understood enough of what I said to offer me a response, even though it was a cryptic one.

"Once upon a time, there was a feather," he told me. "When the feather blew over to the other side of town, it became a feather bed."

After a few quiet moments, I asked him, "What does that mean, Martin?"

"It means things change, doctor, depending on the circumstances."

I still ponder his parable. In one case, the feather is simple and stands alone. In another, the feather multiplies and develops into a dense object with a specific function. Change and transformation occur, but the essence remains the same. Was this what Martin was trying to tell me?

On the other hand, his metaphor may be more akin to the "law of unforeseen consequences," something which my husband, Abe, tends to notice in our daily lives—sometimes more than I wish he would. As we seek to care for our institutionalized sick and infirm, we naturally rely on the way society functions as a whole. We turn to laws, rules, regulations, and financial schemes to build a familiar framework to help us make decisions and practice our skills and knowledge within the nursing home. For all our efforts, however, there is much in the practice of long-term care that we do not—and perhaps cannot—anticipate. What we had envisioned takes shape as something we had not foreseen.

Mirror Images

Betsy Warner makes me think of Martin's feather. She moved in and out of five different facilities in three years. Everywhere she went, she was perceived a little differently than she had been in the last place. With each move her case history grew, yet essentially she remained the same. Her first move from Mission Hill to Serenity Acres took her from a well-run facility with a normal care team to one that was deeply dysfunctional. Although the care she received at the Acres was far different from what it had been at Mission Hill, she retained more or less the same set of problems and the same level of health. Her Parkinson's disease remained under control but for occasional bouts of muscle pain.

Betsy's departure from Mission Hill might be said to illustrate the law of unforeseen consequences. Certainly none of us anticipated the events that led to her quitting the facility. Who could have guessed that Mission Hill's efforts to burnish its image as a "culture change" institution would alienate an entire family?

In theory the idea sounded uncontroversial and even appealing. Mission Hill would improve its hair salon by offering more services, including facials, massage, cosmetic applications, and the offer of beauty and personal hygiene tips, in addition to the usual haircuts and permanent waves. Cammie Faust would remain in charge and oversee the comings and goings of outside contractors, such as the masseuse.

Difficulties arose for familiar reasons. Cammie was outspoken and overbearing. To make matters worse, she was caught up in an unbridled wave of enthusiasm now that she had an amplified role to play and a whole new line of products and services to promote. When Betsy Warner came in for a consultation, she declined anything more than a simple facial. Disappointed, Cammie forgot herself and played doctor again. Reportedly the conversation between the two women deteriorated into something like this:

"You've got big pouches under your eyes, don't you see? Plastic surgery is what you need, and I happen to know a good face man. Here, I'll jot down his number for you."

"No, thank you, Cammie. I don't want surgery; a facial will do."

"All right, but have you given breast reduction any further thought? It would eliminate your back pain. In fact, I'm sure of it."

"Cammie, please. I came in here to relax."

"Well, excuse me for trying. Why you'd want to settle for baggy eyes and enormous boobs is beyond me. Are you afraid of surgery? Well, it's what you need."

Not surprisingly, Betsy did not have a facial after all. With a toss of her head, she left Cammie's shop without a word. It was to her daughters that she voiced her outrage.

Betsy was not just any elderly woman. Still striking, she was a former model, who had for a time reached the great heights of the Ford Agency in New York, and was among the few residents that Mission Hill could count as celebrities of a sort. If Cammie was ignorant of Betsy's claim to fame, perhaps it was because she spent so much time talking herself.

Betsy's daughters were far from pleased. Their mother's vanity had been wounded. Worse still, she had been subjected to unsolicited medical advice in a facility that was supposed to be top-drawer.

"You've got a beautician with rocks in her head," the younger daughter complained to me. "She acts like she's a doctor. Does she get a kickback, do you suppose, from these plastic surgeons she's constantly peddling?"

The Warner women moved quickly to find their mother a new facility. It was unfortunate that they chose Serenity Acres, given its poor care. Yet the choice was fitting, given the importance the women placed on appearances. Once again, those crystal chandeliers in the lobby did their job.

Prima Donna Escapades

Of course no one at the Acres was prepared to treat Betsy like a VIP. In fact, one move alone was enough to brand Betsy a nursing home "hopper." Thus the Acres staff viewed her as a "problem" resident from the outset, which was true at least some of the time. Mrs.

Warner remained as moody and "high-maintenance" as ever. Top-flight attention was not available at the Acres but that did not stop Betsy and her daughters from asking for it.

Yet the Acres thrived on Mrs. Warner, whose inner turmoil complemented the general confusion, even as her mood swings encouraged staff to fight more intently than usual about how to care for her. Amy Gaston was the nurse that fell hardest for Betsy, captivated by the photos of a woman whose face once appeared in the pages of magazines like *Harpers Bazaar* and *Vogue*, and which now hung on the walls of Betsy's small nursing home room, testaments to her once-dazzling career. Amy took her "diva" very seriously, and documented every concern that Betsy or one of her family members raised.

Heidi Schrum thought just the opposite. In her book, Mrs. Warner was an attention-craving faker, who in desperation had turned to illness to retain her self-importance. She refused to give Betsy any medication for pain, even when she asked for it, something she began to do more often, now that she had started to complain of a new stomach ailment. The tug-of-war between the two nurses put Betsy on an uneven keel, to say the least. The Warner women, meanwhile, demanded that their mother be put on a new pain killer, which they had seen advertised in a pharmaceutical journal. Although they had chastised Mission Hill for employing a beautician that often pushed treatments without the knowledge to back them up, they had apparently succumbed to the same temptation.

Maxine Combes, then the facility administrator, referred Betsy's daughters to me. We agreed to meet and discuss their mother's treatment options. A day or two later, I waited in my office for them to arrive. I waited for some time, but no one came.

Before I left the facility, I paid Betsy a visit. She shrugged when I told her that her daughters had failed to show up for our scheduled appointment.

"They have better things to do. I know I did when I was their age."

Betsy seemed bored today and more intent on the state of her fingernails than her stomach. "Where is that manicurist when you need her, anyway?" she wanted to know.   A manicurist at the Acres was a rarity indeed. We did get around to discussing her stomach pain eventually, however, and the possibility of outpatient tests at the local hospital.

"I'll consider it, but I don't want to see him again."

"Who do you mean?"

"Dr. Collins. He's a pill, if you'll pardon the pun."

"You saw him?"

"Yes. He reminded me of my third husband—not a good thing."

"I'm surprised that you went to see him."

"Don't be surprised, doctor. My daughters are my keepers."

Maxine called me shortly afterward. It seemed that Betsy's daughters had lodged a complaint about my lack of involvement in their mother's care. Less informed than I might have been, I explained the situation as best I could.

"They scheduled a meeting with me this morning, but no one showed up."

Far from neglectful, I had just come away from Mrs. Warner with whom I had spent the better part of an hour, discussing what tests to pursue.

"Well, that's part of the problem," Maxine said. "The family is upset about what you said."

"How so?"

Margo Kennedy, it seemed, had told Mrs. Warner's daughters that their mother could not withstand any intensive examination of an exploratory kind. No doubt Margo had reached this conclusion after she had overheard me say, "Betsy Warner has a delicate constitution. She reminds me of that fairy tale—'The Princess and the Pea.'"

Only much later did all that had transpired become clear. Amy Gaston had suggested that Betsy's daughters take their mother to see Abner Collins, the young physician who had left the facility in frustration. Amy accompanied the Warners. She told him that Heidi Schrum's attitude toward Betsy amounted to abuse, and mine to neglect. As she had in the past, she claimed that I was too busy to give my patients the attention they deserved.

Dr. Collins never contacted me, or the facility, to get more information on Betsy's history. Instead, he contacted the state to suggest that she might have been the victim of some mistreatment at the Acres.

In the end a lack of evidence thwarted Dr. Collins' attempt to further blacken the Acres' reputation. Eventually, the Warner family and I had a good meeting, which helped to dispel insinuations that I had somehow neglected their mother.

Betsy had her tests, which revealed nothing out of the ordinary about her stomach. Shortly thereafter, she stopped complaining about pain of any kind. The test results had settled her down, for the moment at least.

As Martin Scanlon said, a feather on one side of town can travel to the other side and become a feather bed. Now I had discovered that the feather bed could travel back in the opposite direction. Once again, it could simply be a feather.

Six
A Doctor's Dilemmas

My days proceed, prospectively in time but retrospectively in spirit—like my scrapbook. Their mundane nature, largely the result of my experience, is overwhelmed by a complex history of emotions. The older I get, the more multifaceted these feelings become. Sometimes I feel defeated, at other times triumphant.

Whenever I question what it means to be a doctor in nursing homes, I am haunted by former patients. Sally Ballard is one of them. In a fleeting second, I am powerless as I imagine her, wheeling through the parking lot, looking for what was not there. What was she thinking as she scrawled graffiti in nail polish on the dementia unit's brand new door? Did she feel ashamed of her actions once she came face to face with the care team, whose members were either too shocked or too thoughtless to try to understand her intentions? My role as her caring physician had eroded badly. Far from an advocate, who might explain my patient's state of mind, I was merely the servant of her insurer, who dictated how I was to treat Sally. She was allowed a pretzel only by virtue of my willingness to oblige the insurance company with extensive documentation.

No one was going to consult me about her inner thoughts, yet I would have liked to understand Sally's intentions as she took her last voyage across the parking lot. Was it freedom she craved, or just a chance to breathe fresh air? Maybe she wanted to exert some sovereignty, to show that she was not controlled entirely by her keepers. Alternatively, and much more simply, her exodus may have been preprogrammed. Maybe instinct took over—no motive, no reason. Her venture out to the asphalt may have been but a last pirouette in her life cycle.

My spirit sinks whenever I witness the predicament of a patient like Sally, and I have seen many patients in similar situations. In their

final efforts to act like human beings, too often they receive nothing
but scorn from irritated staff and even family. Health care institutions have created a slew of safety nets to protect against risks, which
they believe they must assume. The side effect is to stifle the freedom
of choice and dignity of the very people they purportedly serve.

Yet my spirit does lift eventually, as does my sense of hope.
Who knows? I might actually help someone. Sally's last efforts to as-
sert herself did not prolong her life. In a weakened state, her fate was
sealed already. Yet her gumption continues to hearten me even as I
strain to find ways to support the same show of spirit in patients like
her.

What does not dissolve, however, is a sense of weariness, worn
down as I am by the pervasive influence of ancillary employees, not
to mention amateurs, who ride the coattails of medical professionals—and often leave us in the dust.

Do such people help the individual patient? Rarely. Do they
help me to do my job? On occasion. Do they help themselves? Always. As a rule, the relationship between the physician and the quasi-
professional in long-term care facilities is a parasitic one. Admittedly,
a symbiosis may develop sometimes, as we shall see.

An Educational Ordeal

I seldom recall the many years of formal education, which pre-
ceded the career I have today. As a sort of coping mechanism, I treat
this part of my life like a black hole. The lure of becoming a physician
was the gravitational pull, but nine years of postgraduate educational
experience was painful enough to want to suppress. Four years of
medical school, three years of residency, and two years of a fellowship add up to a lot of time to give to a goal—ten percent of my life,
if I live to be ninety; twenty percent at this point. The commitment
meant the surrender of other options. A part of me was lost. Luckily,
I was long married and did not have to also forgo a personal life, as
did so many other medical students.

As any physician will tell you, the commitment to medicine is
more than a matter of time. Medical school entails grueling classes and test after test for two years, followed by two more years of
clinical activity, performed with notorious sleep deprivation. Like in-

dentured servants from another century, we medical students in the 1980s were issued small beds with old sheets to sleep in for a few hours a night, and were otherwise expected to work nearly continuously, that is, about twenty-eight days out of every thirty. In exchange, we paid tuition—an exorbitant amount that annually outstripped the average family income in this country—to attend a midrange school. I am not a fan of medical education as it is taught today, but somehow we did learn. It was painful, and I do question the wisdom of such an archaic system—a "see-one-do-one-teach-one" type of learning that was a structured initiation process more than anything else.

Nearly thirty at the time, I was among the eldest of my peers when I also became pregnant. The combination made me something of an anomaly. To add insult to injury, I rejected mainstream obstetrical practice and chose a nurse-midwife to oversee my pregnancy and delivery at home. This choice, which perhaps one in ten thousand expectant women make in my city, was one I believed in ardently, even though I was probably the only student in my school to make this choice in decades. My reasons were complex and not relevant here, except to note that my peers did not give me a whole lot of support. My age and career put me in a high-risk category, at least from the statistically generic standpoint that they chose to take. My individual health was overlooked in favor of the calculated odds.

Branded as a risk taker, I took personal responsibility for my decision, and vowed not to blame anyone if a perfect outcome did not occur. In fact, I did experience a trouble-free pregnancy, and an easy labor and delivery. Despite the subpar conditions in which she developed, Shira was born a perfectly healthy baby. To this day, the choices that my husband and I made regarding our daughter's birth are viewed by many as outlandish at best, a verdict that tends to remind me of the reaction of nursing home staff to Sally Ballard's bold journey into the parking lot.

Three years of residency in internal medicine followed. For the first time, we students were paid for our work, something noteworthy that we could point to, if a bit wryly, at least those of us who, by then, were in our thirties. Still, the whole period was unpleasant. Residency involved a forty-eight-hour shift with just a catnap or two.

Some new government regulations were put into place to limit our long hours, but there seemed always to be a loophole. We may have gotten an hour more of sleep a week than our predecessors did, but we were painfully tired. There was not much formal teaching, but testing was fairly frequent. Standardized tests at the national level ensured fairness, but of course they were not easy to pass.

Finally, I spent two years as a fellow in geriatrics. The pay was not much better, but an ordinary life style had become an option again. By that time, however, I barely knew what "normal" was. Like a child, I had to learn what people did with their lives. I was grateful to sleep in my own bed every night, just as I am fifteen years later, never having taken the privilege for granted since. Most weekends were free but for the ones when I was on call for emergencies. More important, I had a significant amount of autonomy. I was a bona fide physician and could have a positive impact on others, without sacrificing my own health and sanity.

When my turn came to supervise residents, it gave me great pleasure to exercise this autonomy and treat them quite differently than I and my fellows had been treated, even if my priorities were frowned on. I gave my charges interesting things to do and let them eat and sleep. I gave them time off, too, when they needed it.

At last, I became me—a practicing geriatrician. I felt content, accomplished, and proud. My full-time education was complete, although I would still need to earn continuing medical education credits every year, and take a rigorous recertification exam every decade.

Lately, however, the sense of satisfaction that I take in my professional life has begun to wane. My aspirations to make a positive contribution often seem out of reach. As my story makes clear, I am not disillusioned with medicine. I am disenchanted with how the profession is managed, particularly in my bailiwick of long-term care. I face many hurdles, none of which has anything to do with how I care for my patients. What at times seems insurmountable is not the struggle to treat disease and accept death and debility. It is the circuitous path I am forced to tread to avoid an ever more complicated management system, even as I continue to do all I can to provide good care.

My daughter Shira is quite intent on following in my footsteps and going into medical school—to become a geriatrician at that. She is the same daughter that grew inside me as I spent night after night sleeping in the Spartan hospital call room for a few hours before I would be summoned from sleep to do the menial work of a medical student.

I am proud that my daughter sees me as a role model. Only what should I tell her about her quest to become a physician? The answer, if there is one, is multifaceted. Again, I recall Sally. Out in the parking lot in her wheelchair, she made her last connection with the world outside the nursing home. She experienced some sense of ordinary life at the very end of her own. Yet the nursing home administrators had no choice but to call the corporate office. Risk managers needed to analyze the episode, which was viewed as a grave security violation, and not at all an old woman's breath of fresh air. Should I treat Shira's aspiration in the same way—as a risk to be assessed and managed? Perhaps I should not even attempt to do so myself. I could hire a consultant to do these things for me. On the other hand, I could let destiny preside, along with honesty about the challenges I have experienced. As a risk taker myself, of course, it should come as no surprise that I would not choose to discourage Shira, even if her passion and her effort did not lead to success and satisfaction.

A Struggle to Serve

I have elaborated on my training not to boost my image or to advertise my importance. I abhor titles and the flaunting of status rather than achievement, which to my mind has to do with character and service to others. I have outlined my education to underscore the training and commitment aimed toward a purpose, namely, to do what I want most to do—to give skilled care to the elderly. Instead, as should be clear, I find myself struggling to redirect time away from administrative paperwork and devote it instead to actual hands-on caring and curing. The struggle is a difficult one, even when the care needed is the relatively simple, palliative kind appropriate for someone like Sally. It is as if an invisible force field separates me and my patients, even when we sit right alongside one other.

At the same time, I have seen a real change in attitude over the past fifteen years among patients and their families. The change, unfortunately, is not to the good. My respect for those I serve is not always reciprocated, to say the least. I am treated all too often with discourtesy and sometimes even with threatening and retaliatory behavior, which can leave me distraught.

Faced with the aging process and its attendant problems, many now take a superior, know-it-all attitude. Among the results is an uptick in the number of patients and their families that demand a blank prescription pad with my signature at the bottom—no ifs, ands, or buts. How can my training mean nothing, compared with information that can be found on Google or Wikipedia or television? In fact I feel pressured to do what I know will cause harm. The customer is always right, even if he or she is incorrect, or is misinformed by third parties with a profit motive all their own. One saving grace, at least, is that patients and families are almost always well intentioned. Thus I see it as my job to teach them—or to "unteach" them—where necessary.

Of course it is easy to second-guess the medical professional. Everyone thinks that he or she knows enough about medicine to make a diagnosis. We all have bodies and have experienced illnesses, after all. By contrast, my husband, who is a computer scientist, receives little unsolicited input. Theoretically, a client of his might be daft enough to say, "Abe, I want you to use Einstein's theory of relativity to tell me why my computer is not working today. I demand an explanation, or I'll fire you."

Such an absurd demand would be akin to what I hear all the time: "Dr. Silber, I want you to arrange a total body MRI for my mother (who happens to be 104 years old) and find out why she's tired. If you won't, I'll get another doctor."

In short, the caring professions now endure the worst of many worlds—the fantastic demands made by disgruntled consumers, the restrictions imposed by self-serving regulators, and the Byzantine consequences that arise from trying to accommodate the competing and skewed interests of pharmaceutical companies, hospitals, nursing home corporate offices, and insurance companies. I may feel aggravated and demoralized, but the real brunt is borne by the ill patient and the dying elder.

Ancillary but Everywhere

It is ancillary professionals that create an invisible force field that separates a physician from a patient, even if these colleagues of mine are largely oblivious to the obstructive role they play as we confer day-to-day. Typically, they are housekeepers, practical nurses, billing representatives, marketing persons, lawyers, and insurance representatives. Ironically, it is to their needs, and not to those of my patients, that I spend most of my days catering. It is also to their opinions that I must listen, with regard to things that they know little about, or with regard to motives that have more to do with profit and job security than with health care and patients' well-being.

The Billing Consultant. Consider Tabitha Jenkins, for example, who works as a billing consultant to physicians. Tabitha is a lovely young lady of about twenty-two with a high school degree, who knows billing codes, diagnosis codes, and how to get paid for them. I met her one day to ensure that my documentation was acceptable to insurance companies in case I was audited; nearly everyone is, eventually. Although expert at medical records, Tabitha knows nothing about medicine itself and has no medical education. She does not pretend to.

I handed her one of my progress notes from a patient visit. She compared my notes against a computerized template, cut and pasted a few items, and made a few suggestions. Presto, I would get paid thirty-three percent more from the insurance companies just by using a new billing code with the same information. Tabitha also told me that if I documented five to eight body systems during my exams, instead of three to five, I would be paid fifty percent more. Furthermore, Medicare was about to cut reimbursement, she said. I would have to improve the way that I documented my activities if wanted to make the same living. I guess God exists after all, I thought, if in the form of a billing consultant.

The more extensively I document a patient's care, the more I am paid. The more I know as a practitioner, however, has no bearing. The pay rate is fixed, based on a formula in which there is no place for my added knowledge and skill. The bottom line: I would be better off financially were I to take lessons from Tabitha than to pursue continuing medical education, unless I were to study insurance guidelines.

Once again, my thoughts returned to the grueling training that I had undergone to enter my career, and I began to feel as undermined as I do when patients take Google's word over mine when it comes to their diagnoses and treatment. To game insurance companies with the right choice of words was not why I had spent sleepless nights on hospital rotation. On the surface it might have appeared innocent enough. In the long run, however, to shape a medical practice with a word game played to reap the maximum monetary return would, I felt, lead me farther afield from the effort and thought required to provide quality care. If there is someone that can offer you a simple answer to a complex problem—beware. I decided to stick to my own choice of words and put more effort into finding new ways to improve care.

The Preauthorization Representative. The preauthorization rep is a relative newcomer to the nursing home world. Not so long ago, preauthorization from an insurance company was required only to request coverage for complex and expensive medical tests, or to prescribe medications considered exotic. Today, especially with the onset of Medicare Part D, even very common medications, such as iron supplements, vitamins, and simple analgesics, need to be preauthorized. In addition to procedures and medications, time spent in a hospital or nursing facility needs to be justified. Does the representative, who will decide whether or not to preauthorize an extra day in the hospital, realize, for example, that the ninety-nine-year-old woman in question has no family and nowhere else to go ? Will she be discharged to a homeless shelter? The answer: Most preauthorization nurses do not know and presumably do not care. They represent an insurance company, and the goal is to make money.

I make it a point to seek preauthorization by cell phone during long commutes, as the process tends to be a long one. Just to get someone to answer my call usually takes ten minutes, and I must have to hand the patient's identification number, or my request will be doomed from the start. I call prepared, however, and a data entry clerk with a high school degree and no medical training reads me a list of questions off a computer screen. If I answer enough questions correctly, I will win the prize of preauthorization and be free to prescribe what I had already determined was medically warranted. If not, I will have the right to contest the decision, as long as I meet another set of requirements.

If I decide to contest, I must speak to a nurse, who uses a somewhat more complex set of computer-generated questions. Yet I will be painfully aware of his or her lack of knowledge, given that most preauthorization nurses cannot pronounce many of the words on the screen. As they massacre the medical terms, I doubt that they understand the questions they ask. Sometimes they resort to spelling the words. The botched transposition of syllables and insertion of vowels make me recall the spelling error that led to the faulty diagnosis used to explain Mrs. Arbenz's death.

What is my recourse if I do not succeed the second time? I can ask for a physician's review. (Is the patient dead yet? Has the quickly growing cancer progressed to the point that there are no treatment options? Perhaps.) Contact with a doctor is not that easy, nor that forthcoming. I name two or three windows of time when I can be reached and a phone number for him or her to call me. At least we will move beyond the faltering parroting of foreign phrases at a computer: A real dialog will take place between me and the reviewing physician. Still, the decision often will have been made before our phone conversation occurs. I am obliged to be polite. If I complain too much, I may be taken off the insurance panel altogether for noncompliance with suggested "guidelines." Who makes the guidelines? The insurance company, of course.

It used to be that when I made an initial call for preauthorization, I would speak to a different representative every time. Amid the initial chaos of Medicare part D, however, I had to call so often that a young lady named Polly answered at least five times. Could Polly be my new telephone psychotherapist? We did achieve enough familiarity that I felt I could begin to ask her "unauthorized questions." How did she get this job? What were her qualifications, given that she was

the first person to decide whether my residents would be able to undergo a test or begin to take a drug that a medical examination and
assessment had deemed advisable.

Fresh out of high school, Polly had started her career working
for a telephone market survey clearinghouse. Next, she worked for
the mail order division of a large retailer. Finally, she landed this great
job. The advantages? The work was not seasonal and the pay better
and, of course, she had good benefits—she worked for an insurance
company after all.

I am left to wonder whether the surge in preauthorization
screening, and thus in second-guessing, will alter the type of person
that enters the field of medicine. Polly, for example, might decide to
go to medical school, not because she was interested in science, but
because she knew how to work the system and would want to earn a
good living as a physician preauthorization agent. Such a new subspe-
cialty might indeed flourish as an insurance company's best line of
defense. A physician that handled initial preauthorization requests
would cost more to employ than a data entry clerk. The savings, however, associated with better articulated reasons to deny coverage, and
to discourage reviews of such decisions, presumably would more than
make up the difference.

The Marketing Representative. Another important player in
nursing home care is the marketing representative, such as Sharon
Suttles, who ably fills that role for GeriMed, the group of geriatricians with whom I practice. Sharon and I are a real team. She uses her
creativity and interpersonal skills as an experienced social worker to
market what I hope is an excellent product—my medical skills—and
she leaves the medicine to me. If she makes a recommendation now
and then about my practice, I suppose I do the same about hers.

With a master's degree in social work, Sharon is bright, organized, and energetic, and meets with me periodically to discuss any
issues or problems that arise regarding the facilities I serve, whether
on their end or on mine. She also helps me find new facilities in which
to work or to house some of my patients, if I am interested. Likewise,
I promote the hospital system that employs her, which I do believe
provides high-quality care.

I have no ethical misgivings with marketing and selling medical care, pharmaceuticals, and medical testing per se. What I do take issue with—and which occurs frequently today—is to put the marketing ahead of the product. In fact, it is not unheard of for potential medical services to be marketed before they exist. In my opinion, marketing should not be done unless the product is worthy. Yet it is commonplace to promote an inferior or a marginally useful one, as Serenity Acres does all the time.

The Pharmaceutical Representative. Harry Simon is one of the few pharmaceutical representatives whom I have met over the years that I actually like. Every few months we meet for coffee. These get-togethers are mutually advantageous. I learn more about the drug company through the eyes of an insider. He, meanwhile, earns points with his higher-ups for getting some face time with a real doctor.

In short, Harry is in sales. He is no different than a car salesman, a computer salesman, or a clothing salesman. He is not successful unless he sells. Whether his product is good, bad, or indifferent, Harry must convince us that it is desirable, will not cause patients to die prematurely, and should warrant coverage by insurance providers. Because reality is largely a matter of how we perceive—and what we believe—Harry retains a good shot at success.

Many of us physicians, in fact, feel bullied by drug reps. They drain time from days that are already too short. They are aggressive and provide little useful information. On occasion they have greeted me at the entrance to a long-term facility with a box of doughnuts in hand.

"I heard that you were in the area, Dr. Silber. Do you have a moment for me?"

Do I have a choice without being terribly rude? I already know that the "moment" will involve a pitch: Surely I have resident patients that need the latest cure?

Physicians do not practice in a vacuum. Usually, we are at least loosely associated with certain hospitals or insurance plans. Hospitals and pharmacies often enjoy rebates and other discounts associated with the use of a sole vendor and the bundling of certain pharmaceutical products. Only physicians can do the prescribing, but can we be coerced into doing so? Of course.

Hospital managers often ask me to make myself available to their pharmaceutical representatives, because the companies they represent "give themselves to our hospitals," in the way of donated money and services. What this generosity really amounts to is a negotiated settlement between a given hospital and a pharmaceutical company. The drug reps, whom I am expected to make nice with, will steer me to the preferred products. If I decline to use them, it is possible that the hospitals will look for other physicians that will.

Likewise, insurance companies may create clinical guidelines on a particular illness. These guidelines can be unduly influenced—not by medical science—but by the marketing campaigns of pharmaceutical companies as well as other special interest groups. Such guidelines may amount to little more than the promotion of a certain medication, treatment, or test. Again, the realities of medical practice may not align with scientific facts. The perception of what is true is what matters most—like Gospel.

Theoretically, of course, doctors are completely free to decide whether or not to follow such treatment guidelines. In fact, however, we are coerced into compliance: We are threatened with expulsion from the market otherwise. We may even be sued, as such guidelines have come to be accepted as standards of care through the varied influences of disease advocacy groups, drug manufacturers, hospitals, and even fellow physicians. Suffice it to say, few of these guidelines are based on pure, unadulterated fact. Regardless of their real worth, however, physicians are strongly urged to follow them to guard against legal action. Thus if we wish to continue to work as physicians, we must go along with the current system. Who controls the caring profession now? Certainly not physicians, as I and my colleagues are only too well aware.

The Lawyer. Medical practice today is intertwined with the practice of law. Thus attorneys count among the ancillary professionals with whom I deal on a regular basis. John Siddle is one of them. I have worked with John on several cases involving charges of negligence, and served as an expert analyst. As a fairly typical example, the two of us met to discuss my initial thoughts after I had received in the mail and reviewed about fifty pounds worth of charts from the attorney for a deceased patient whose family alleged inappropriate care. The case, although typical, disturbed me. To claim, as this family did, that a nursing home and its staff must provide an absolute guarantee against accidents involving incontinence and physical falls is unrealistic and indeed such a case on its face is usually without merit unless evidence is produced of actual carelessness or neglect.

When first approached to act as an expert reviewer in the depositions of such cases, I was intrigued. Perhaps I could be of genuine assistance and help some of my colleagues extricate themselves in an era of frivolous litigation. Of course, the extra income would not hurt, either. I received a hefty fee, as I was one of the few fellowship-trained geriatricians in town with the requisite experience. In short order, however, I came to realize that no one really wanted my expert opinion. I was wanted only if I would say the right thing, not the true thing. I was the expert, but my opinion was written for me.

Not so long ago, a colleague's practice and reputation were on the line. My deposition, which I had painstakingly written, was recast entirely to conform to a corporate template. The result reminded me of the way in which Tabitha Jenkins, the billing specialist, had tried to upgrade my fees with a few adjustments to a preprogrammed set of codes in her computer.

What do these various folks need me for, I am left to wonder, except to give their endeavors some sort of phony seal of approval? Forced into the role of front woman, I feel more like a fraud than a physician.

The disappointment I experienced as a medical expert in lawsuits quickly gave way to the realization that the desired outcome (winning) was all that mattered, not how we got there. Ironically, I found myself respecting the legal profession for that attitude. Thinking about the attorney's goals, I wondered about my own. What were my main concerns as a practicing physician? There were not to be sued, not to get my charts audited, to get my malpractice insurance renewed, to get insurance companies to approve my charges, and to get my prescriptions for drugs pre-approved quickly. I cannot say I am proud that these are the first goals that come to mind. The true purposes of the practice of medicine, after all, are to promote health, extend the life span, treat illness, and offer a better quality of life. None of the goals that I stated above helps me fulfill my true purposes. In fact, they can stand squarely in the way.

Most perplexing is that we physicians defer on a daily basis to ancillary professionals, who not only are less informed than we are about medicine but who also have agendas contradictory to its basic tenets. Medical care, in its true and fullest forms of expression, is constrained within the confines that other people create to carry out their own functions.

A Daughter Does Harm

Sometimes I have managed to escape such confines. When I have, it has largely been the circumstances and the outlook of my patients that have permitted me to be the doctor that I had always dreamed of being and had studied so hard to become. Imogene MacDowell was one of these patients. If teachers have pets, so do doctors. Imogene was mine. A creative and industrious person, she made her own greeting cards and sent them to every resident in her independent living facility, as well as to many others of her acquaintance. Each card was unique and made clever and artistic use of pictures clipped from the magazines that Imogene subscribed to over the years. I have received quite a few of these cards myself, and have tucked them away for safekeeping.

I first met Imogene on the lovely grounds that surround Mission Hill. She lived on her own, she proudly told me, in a one-bedroom apartment adjacent to the nursing home. Our casual conversations led to a friendly rapport and eventually to my taking her on as a patient on an informal basis. Although I documented my visits, I did not bill her insurance company, as her policy would cover but a tiny portion of my fee for home visits, and she could not afford to pay me herself.

Given her aversion to nursing homes, it was fortunate that institutionalization was not in the offing. A physical exam showed that she had arthritis, mild hypertension, and a few other nonlife-threatening problems, which I relegate to the minor status of "important nuisances." I began to call on her about once a month, as much to socialize as to check up on her health. Each time, Imogene had a list of problems for me—usually about ten—neatly written on a piece of lined paper.

Imogene's questions, as I soon learned, were predicated on her strong desire to remain in the apartment in which she lived independently and where she had control over most aspects of her daily life. Always she remained acutely aware that, on the other side of the fence, lay the nursing home facility, where she would have far less say. Her day-to-day rituals clearly were designed (whether consciously or instinctively) to make sure that she would stay on the side that she preferred. I, too, was part of Imogene's designs to stay on that right side. She placed her hope in me. In my way, I placed my hope in her also. Imogene's independent living status gave me more freedom to practice medicine than I usually had. I enjoyed it. Without the strictures of the care plan and the care team and the host of ancillary professionals to answer to, I sensed no barrier between us. Imogene and I had a completely open patient-doctor rapport.

After I answered all of Imogene's questions, which actually did not take long, she would ask about my family. Sometime I would bring along a scrapbook of mine for her to look at, or some photos. I thought of us as friends. Still, she always had her list of questions ready for me when I came. Most of them were just variations on the same themes. A typical list would read like the following one:

1. My leg swells in the afternoon. What should I do?
2. I heard ginkgo is good for memory. Should I try it?
3. May I take two aspirins a day if I have a headache?
4. I feel bloated when I eat pumpkin pie.
5. Why are my sinuses worse in the spring?
6. May I take my vitamin three times a day? It makes me feel better.
7. How much should I walk a day?
8. My left hip hurts for ten minutes every time I go to sleep at night.
9. I am stiff in the morning. Do I need a knee replacement?
10. When can I see you again?

Something of a medical researcher, Imogene pored over the *Readers' Digest Guide to Vitamins, Minerals and Supplements (Medical Guide)*, among other resources. Although she did not know how to "surf the net," her daughter, Darla, did. Imogene was very proud of her daughter and boasted about her computer expertise.

On occasion, Imogene's compulsiveness about her health would escalate. Now and then she would telephone between visits with another list of ten questions. Sometimes she would call me three times a day. She would call her daughter even more frequently and sometimes throughout the night. Her stomach hurt on the left and then on the right. Her heel itched or her throat hurt.

After a particularly disruptive night during which Imogene had called twelve times, her daughter had had enough. Darla called me the following morning and asked me to prescribe an antibiotic for Imogene. Problem was, an antibiotic was completely inappropriate and counter to every scientific and medical guideline, not to mention all common sense. In fact, inappropriate antibiotic use was contraindicated in her case and could have caused harm. I sat down with Imogene and told her why I did not think that an antibiotic was advisable. She seemed satisfied with my explanation and said that she simply wanted to do what was best.

Darla did not accept my reasoning, however. After I said no to the antibiotic, she asked me to stop treating her mother. My professional manners intact, I accepted her decision. Privately, I was cut to the quick. Imogene disappeared from my life, and I heard nothing more about her until Wendy Perkins hailed me in the hallway.

What the Housekeeper Knew

Wendy was a housekeeper at the Acres. She had the spirit of a young country girl, although her prematurely wrinkled skin from years of farming under the intense sun made her age difficult to determine. I knew her fairly well—well enough, in fact, to try and avoid her. As sweet and kind as Wendy was, she loved to talk. Embarrassingly, my attempt to slip by her in the busy corridor did not work. I accepted my fate and surrendered to what would be longwinded stories about her family woes. Instead, she surprised me.

"Do you remember Imogene MacDowell?"

Wendy's simple question startled me. Almost a year had passed since I had seen Imogene. I had resisted the temptation to visit her apartment complex near Mission Hill, but I had hoped I might see her on the grounds, where we first met. I never did see her out for a stroll, however, and it crossed my mind more than once that Imogene might have passed.

"She's alive then?"

"Yes, but she's not well."

I barely listened to how Wendy was acquainted with Imogene—something tiresomely complicated about her daughter's ex-husband's live-in boyfriend being related to Wendy's sister-in-law. In any event, somehow my name had come up in conversation this morning, and Imogene learned that I was still in practice, something that surprised her. Apparently, Darla had told Imogene otherwise.

"She's not at all well," Wendy repeated. "Her doctor put her on an antibiotic about a year ago for a reason nobody can figure out. Would you have done that?"

Without waiting for an answer, Wendy continued. "Poor Imogene has had nothing but trouble ever since." After she started taking the medicine, Imogene developed severe diarrhea, related to the treatment. On the way to the toilet, she fell and was not found until about twelve hours later, when she did not show up for breakfast, as she usually did, at the assisted-living facility's communal dining room. She was hospitalized for the fall and dehydration.

How hard that must have been on her, I thought, knowing how uncomfortable Imogene was with institutions like hospitals. She returned home quickly, which caused her daughter some concern. Although Imogene was no doubt happy to leave the hospital, she probably remained fixated on her health as well. If Darla had not demanded a full medical workup, perhaps Imogene would have done so herself. In any case, she underwent an angiogram and developed an acute reaction to the dye used in the procedure from which she nearly died. Although the experience was harrowing for both mother and daughter, neither could resist further inquiry. Why did Imogene have an allergic reaction to the dye?

Darla spent hours on the Internet, pursuing every diagnosis and potential intervention. Imogene underwent blood test after blood test, procedure after procedure. Nothing seemed wrong until one day a doctor did find a small lesion on an artery in her neck. Perhaps her artery was dilated. If so, there was a possibility, albeit a highly remote one, the doctor said, that Imogene could be at greater risk for a stroke. Imogene underwent a procedure to excise the lesion. Unfortunately, she had a stroke during the procedure. The hospitalization that followed was complicated. Imogene was on a feeding tube and could not walk, Wendy said. Assisted living was out of the question, and Mission Hill had no vacancies at the time. Given the urgency of the situation, Darla had moved her mother into the Serenity Acres nursing home.

"She's in Room 122," Wendy said.

Shocked, I also felt terribly sad. Here was Wendy telling me that Imogene was right here, not more than a few doors away, a resident in a nursing home, a fate that she had so hoped to avoid. Poor Imogene. When it came to her independence, she had strayed over to the wrong side of the fence.

Yet I have to admit I was angry too. Here was another instance in which medical care was manipulated by a person that had no real understanding of medicine. At the root of so much unnecessary suffering lay the impatience and irritation of a daughter, who was sick of her mother's complaints yet had put her through the mill for a definitive diagnosis. Why was Imogene in this room now and not living independently back in her own apartment near Mission Hill? Because her daughter wanted a medical cure to avoid being called in the middle of the night by her lonely and scared mother. Her search for a cure led to a cascade of unfortunate events I could have easily foretold. But who was I? Merely a medical professional, who had seen similar motivations lead to similar outcomes way too many times. As far as Darla was concerned, however, her mother was that one in a million to whom the ordinary, the expected, and the inevitable did not apply.

Wendy disturbed me further with her own observations. "Sorry, if I sound disrespectful, Dr. Silber, but what are these doctors thinking? I can tell you why Imogene fell. Imogene needed to get to the toilet in a hurry. She is an old tired lady and has had many children. Her private parts are loose—you know what I mean—she wears a pad. Imogene is a proud woman, you know—she wouldn't want to soil her panties. Do we need a medical test for that?"

I had to agree. What are we thinking? Let's just help Imogene to the commode. Well, none of us gets paid for that. And what about the risk? If we helped her, Imogene could fall.

"I hear that she moves so little that she suffers from bedsores. She doesn't have much to say for herself. Her mood is very low. Maybe you could help her, doctor."

"No, I don't think so," I said. "Imogene's daughter was very firm. She no longer wants me to see her mother as a patient."

"Oh, I think she's changed her mind by now," Wendy said.

After our conversation, I moved down the corridor until I came to Room 122. At the door, I peeked inside. There she was—barely recognizable—but still Imogene. Seated in a wheelchair, she did not see me, bent as she was over a small notebook on her lap in which she was scribbling. Perhaps she was making a list of questions for her current physician? Or perhaps she was writing a birthday greeting? That was what I preferred to think. I would have hesitated to go in and disturb her, even if I had not felt the need to talk to Darla first.

Seven
Shades of Care

One thing about nursing homes is that every resident's room has a past. People come and go, sometimes at a phenomenal rate. Lives culminate, sucked in and packed with the density and pull of a time warp. Given each room's intricate emotional history, it is no wonder that I often hesitate on the threshold. It is hard to concentrate on the person right in front of me when, just the week before, I cried as a resident died in that same bed, or a year ago, I had enjoyed a good laugh with a resident that has since gone home.

I am haunted by room décor. The items that patients bring from their own homes often tell me volumes about their personalities and the kind of lives that they have led. If I were to come to live in one of these rooms, what I would I bring? I have a large home. How would I choose and discard objects from a lifetime?

The renovations that nursing home corporations tend to approve every few years serve marketing purposes, and yet a facelift on a sagging image also helps to dim the past. Still, a fresh coat of paint and new pictures on the walls can only do so much. Memories do persist in these rooms where people live out their final days. Imogene MacDowell's room was no exception.

The Many Lives of Room 122

Before she arrived in Room 122, it was home to two women patients of mine—Monica, a ninety-seven-year-old Catholic nun, who constantly feared that she would gain weight and look fat, and Dottie, the only black person in the facility, who used her electric wheelchair to get around and flirt with certain men that caught her eye. She courted her prospective beaus by giving them the extra single-serve jams and jellies from her breakfast trays. Once things were getting serious, she would bestow on her latest boyfriend one of the ceramic figurines, which she had made in the craft room. Neither senile nor shallow, Dottie was able to enjoy genuinely caring and affectionate relationships. Although age and death cut short some of her romances, she managed to have several that appeared to run quite deep.

Once when Dottie was laid up with cellulitis and was too weak to use her wheelchair, Monica took me aside. "I know you'll do all you can for her medically, but could you do something else?"

"And what would that be?" I asked.

"Could you please find Bob Chatfield? It would brighten her day if she could see him."

Bob, I did not need to be told, was Dottie's latest love.

Before these ladies inhabited Room 122, the Cottrells lived there. Husband and wife, each was ninety-five years old. They were the parents of Carol Sue Redmon, a nursing supervisor at Mission Hill and a friend of mine. Millicent Cottrell had a sweet nature and perfect manners. Dave Cottrell was cantankerous, obstinate, and rude when he felt he needed to be, having relied on these same traits to run a large and successful corporation for some forty years. He occupied himself largely by dreaming up ways to create a new business from inside the nursing home.

"An incompetent, money-hungry scoundrel," was what he called Maxine, who had run the Acres as its administrator for many years. He was probably half-right, as Maxine had kept the facility running in the black—always—even during rough times.

Mr. Cottrell had taken up smoking in his nineties. Once, in this very room, he decided to indulge his new habit and then fell asleep in his armchair. Fortunately, a passing nurse was able to douse the fire that his burning cigarette had set to the newspaper that he had left on an adjacent table. Maxine responded with a prohibition against smoking anywhere inside the facility. Far from contrite, Dave raged against her more. He deliberately passed intestinal gas to provoke people, particularly those whom he did not much care for, and Maxine was a prime target.

He believed, I suppose, that he had nothing left to lose. After all, he was very old, living in a nursing home, and spending his hard-earned fortune on subpar care. What he feared most, he told me, was that eventually his money would be gone. To depend on public assistance would be for him the worst indignity of the many that he and his wife already had endured.

Before the Cottrells lived in Room 122, Erich Nelsen did. In his mid-eighties, he was moved off the dementia ward and placed under hospice care. Diagnosed with end-stage Alzheimer's disease, he had not eaten for two weeks. His family, all of whom were resigned to the fact that he was passing, gathered often in Room 122. Mr. Nelsen had been through several crises, which for him and his extended family were like rehearsals for his death; all were ready for the real thing. When I entered the room to ask if anyone had any questions, people were actually joking and laughing with each other. Everyone was appreciative and gracious, and they thanked me for caring for Dad, who to their minds had passed away long ago.

At the time I was working on an art project at home that called for lots of unshelled nuts. I had searched through every grocery in the city but found none. It was February at the time, and it looked like I would have to wait until November, when the stores usually got unshelled nuts in again for the holidays. As I turned to leave Room 122, I caught sight of the table in the far corner on which Mr. Nelsen's family had set out some food, including just what I had been looking for—nuts—pecans, walnuts, Brazil nuts, almonds, and every one of them inside its very own shell. I was ashamed. A man was dying, with his family at his bedside, and all I could think of was how much I coveted that bowl on the back table.

I also recall Hope Brown, a long-time patient of mine, who passed away in this room. As she was dying, my eyes glanced at the box of cookies by her bedside. My family used to eat the same brand all the time. Not anymore.

Would Betsy Warner ever live in this room? It was possible, even though she appeared to be on a quest for the holy grail of nursing homes. Still, she might well settle down here eventually. If she ever did move into Room 122, the childhood photos of her daughters in pinafores would look perfect on the shelf near the window.

Mr. Storage Closet

For a time I had no patients in Room 122 at all. As I passed by one day, I glanced up, expecting to see an empty slot for the nameplate, which, by regulation, must appear outside the door of every resident. Only the brass slot was not empty. Storage Closet, the label read, which stopped me in my tracks. Had a person been admitted and assigned to the room without my knowledge? Could someone actually have such a name? Silly as it might sound, that second question did cross my mind, if fleetingly, as I peeked inside the room. From the threshold, I saw nothing but two stripped beds, some old supplies, and a large stock of new disposable undergarments. To find that I had one less patient to attend was fine, especially as the respite would not last. Yes, the room was being used for storage, but it would be transformed into a two-bed suite in a flash once the census was up again. Meanwhile, the remnants of many lives remained—not only in the room's shadows but also in the labeled charts of former inhabitants retained in facility files.

These charts led to tragicomedy when a new patient, Mr. Parsons, was admitted to the facility right before a shift change. Patty King, who was just coming off duty as nursing supervisor, was eager to leave for the day. She had a date with Alan Barton, the head of maintenance who, in his characteristically loudmouthed way, told her to hurry it up and leave the rest to her relief.

A colorful character, Alan was for all intents and purposes an honorary member of the Acres' care team. He actively participated in morning meetings where nursing staff discussed resident care. Much like Cammie, the beautician at Mission Hill, Alan tended to see himself as an unofficial expert on medicine—a sort of physician-by-proxy. I suppose that, since I use a sink to wash my hands, I could profess to be a plumber. The truth is, of course, that Alan does not know how to diagnose and treat congestive heart failure, and I do not know how to fix a faucet. Yet the general apathy and cynicism of the nursing staff at the Acres created a vacuum into which someone like Alan could step. He who yelled loudest and was the most obnoxious held sway over team meetings. Soon he was seen as an unofficial expert on nearly everything.

Looking forward to their night out, Patty grabbed a chart labeled Room Number 122 and put the new patient's admission paperwork inside. Per Alan's instructions, she left the rest of the admissions tasks for the nursing supervisor about to come on duty.

Her relief was an agency nurse. Usually temporary staff did a poor job but not Arnie Valentine. She had supervised the nursing staff at the Acres several times in the past year and was competent and eager to perform her duties. A Filipino, she had worked as a nurse in the United States for about five years and had been a physician in her native country. Although she claimed to be ill prepared to pass the boards required to practice medicine here, my impression was that she certainly could have passed, had a lack of confidence and perhaps fatigue not stood in the way. In any case, Arnie was heartily disliked at the Acres, precisely because she was punctual, devoted, and careful. A job well done only made everyone else look bad. Besides, her modesty and humility could be annoying.

Perhaps it was dislike, or else an embarrassed sort of evasion, that led Patty to assure Arnie that most all of the work had been completed on the new admission, and the resident was doing well. In any event Arnie turned her attention to other pressing problems that night, including the administration of patient medications on the Peach Unit, where the treatment nurse, Heidi Schrum, had once again walked off the job.

In the meantime, Alan and Patty had gone out to a bar, drank quite a bit, and gotten into a fight. Angry with each other, they cut short their date, and Patty dropped Alan back at the facility, where his car was parked. Alan, who already had been arrested for driving under the influence, knew better than to go home. Instead he let himself into the facility and headed for Room 122 to sleep.

A half-hour later, Arnie got a call from the floor nurse. Mr. Parsons, the new admission, was not doing well. From the deserted nurses' station, Arnie grabbed the chart that Patty had prepared and headed to Room 122. There she did an assessment on the nearly comatose Alan, who was too intoxicated to protest.

Meanwhile, the floor nurse had grown frantic. Where was Arnie? Mr. Parsons was failing.

How quickly events transpired.

Within ten minutes, Mr. Parsons died.

Within twelve hours, the floor nurse kept her secret vow and called the nursing board to complain about Arnie's absence at a critical moment. That she had a grudge against Arnie was well known, and clearly she welcomed the chance to badmouth her. I suspect that, like Patty, she resented Arnie's competence and strong work ethic. Whatever her accusations, the floor nurse was persuasive. The agency declined to use Arnie again, effectively putting an end to her career as a nurse.

Within a day's time, Room 122 went from being a storage closet to the final home of one dying patient, at least on paper. Simultaneously, it had served as the crash pad of an intoxicated employee. Now, lo and behold, the space was home to Imogene.

No wonder I paused outside the door.

Alan Barton, meanwhile, got a raise—the reward of expediency if also ingenuity—on the part of Maxine Combes, that is. Ever adept at keeping up appearances, she had persuaded the corporate office to embrace the "universal worker" principle as a way to smooth over the fact that the admissions paperwork on the deceased Mr. Parsons was mislabeled and incomplete. As an industry trend, the principle permits efficiencies. No longer limited to the scope of one job description, nursing home staff members perform any number of interchangeable daily living tasks, including serving meals, performing light housekeeping, doing laundry, and even filing. Thus the scope of Alan's job expanded beyond maintenance to include help at the nurses' station, and he became a part-time unit clerk. Among other things, he completed the admission paperwork on Mr. Parsons and corrected the label on his file.

Trial by Patient

Not long after I paid my secret visit to Imogene, I received a call from her daughter, Darla. Would I consider taking Mom as a patient again? Of course I would. How could I say no to my favorite elder? Imogene would be a welcome reprieve, given my willingness to take on difficult patients. I have built a thriving practice on my colleagues' rejects, I sometimes joke privately. Job security is doing the job that no one else wants to do.

I have never turned down anyone that has asked me to be his or her physician. My open door policy does not mean, however, that I cater to my patients' every whim. There is a line that I will not cross. Tara Duran taught me that.

Tara was probably the most difficult patient that I have ever agreed to see. Even the staff at the Acres, that notoriously world-weary bunch, took the trouble to warn me that Tara was a tough case. I was to be not the second, nor the third, but the fourth physician to oversee her case during the nine months that she lived at the facility.

I laughed off any concern, as I always seemed to manage, and met my new patient in her room a few days later.

On her door she had pasted a sign: "Enter at your own risk." Inside, the walls were decorated with pictures from fashion magazines; mostly thin women with red hair like hers. Later I would look at some of her photo albums, piled in high stacks everywhere. The pictures inside were candid shots of staff members and of residents. Some of these photos were humorous, whereas others were humiliating. Tara freely admitted that she had not asked for her subjects' consent. I am not sure what her motivation was. She had boxes and boxes of notebooks and paper, most of which were unused. She also had stashes of food—mostly boxes of cereal, bags of chips, and single-serve peanut butter from the kitchen—and all of it scattered everywhere, including the floor and on her bed. Tara was an amateur artist. A few of her sketches taped to the walls showed signs of an offbeat talent. Yet she spent little time drawing. Usually she was wasted on drugs.

Fervently, I took on her case. I may not be able to save many lives, given that I care mostly for the dying and the chronically ill, but I do pride myself on being able to help a difficult patient to cope a bit better with life. Tara was very ill. She had end-stage renal disease and depended on hemodialysis. Her complex medical problems, however, were the easy ones to address. The far bigger challenges were a manipulative personality disorder, coupled with a drug addiction that she had acquired over the years to deal with the misery of dismal social skills.

Under forty, chronic medical illness had aged her prematurely. Her hair had thinned, and so had her skin, which was covered with multiple bruises. She had the wrinkles of a much older woman, as well as the stooped posture and atrophied muscles. Yet her underlying physical makeup suggested that she would have been a beautiful woman under other circumstances.

Our first few visits were uneventful as we got acquainted. Tara spoke of her dream of going to specialists at the Mayo Clinic and the Cleveland Clinic to have back surgery to relieve her chronic pain. Or perhaps she would go to Chicago or Los Angeles. In the meantime, could I increase her pain medications?

I fended off the request, saying that I needed to review her records first. In this way, I bought myself some time to strategize. Already it was clear that Tara did not want me and my help as a physician. What she really wanted was a drug dealer. Only she was out of cash, and Medicaid would have to do.

As it was, Tara did pretty well for herself. She had prescriptions for mega-doses of pain medications, which she received intravenously every three hours. Yet she exhibited none of the clinical signs of physical pain, such as limited function, facial grimacing, elevated blood pressure, and restlessness. What she exhibited instead were the signs of psychological pain, as well as the anxiety, lethargy, and anorexia, associated with the drug addict. Frantic for her fix, she would lie to me and try to manipulate her way into larger doses. If the nurse was one second late to arrive and administer the drugs, Tara would contact the supervisor.

Our honeymoon, dubious as it had been, was over. Tara began to destroy with petty harassment any chance of a rapport between us.

"You never listen to me," she would wail, or "How would you know anything about me? You hardly spend any time with me."

In fact, I spent much more time with her than I did with most residents. When she knew that I was in the building and had not come to see her, she would go out to the nurses' station to announce that she had just had a seizure and needed to be evaluated. It is nearly impossible to have a seizure, get up on one's own, and talk about it without serious injury. As a matter of fact, Tara's serious medical problems—and she had many—were under control at that point. Her drug addiction stood out starkly as the source of the pain that was most alive in her.

"I don't want this type of life," she would scream sometimes, and it was heartrending to see this young woman trapped in so much agony. Yet it was an agony that did not keep her from being sly and, frankly, on the make.

"You write about me in my chart without actually seeing me," she began to wrongly accuse.

Insurance covered only one visit a month, but because I was concerned about her, I saw her more often, although I did not bill for my extra visits. Being an avid reader of her own chart, she was aware of the notes that I had written, just as she was aware of my several visits. What was she up to?

I began to see Tara with a nurse present. I would document my visit, and the nurse would document my visit. If Tara still wanted to claim that I wrote notes about phantom assessments, she would have to say that we were both lying. After all the sturm und drang, I would receive about thirty dollars for my trouble. What hurt, of course, was the sense that Tara had become a foe.

Attempts to help with her drug addiction were complicated by her genuine need for some narcotic medications to ease the real pain she suffered from her physical disease. I sent her to a pain clinic. After several visits there, the clinic's team told her that she was not allowed to return, as she was noncompliant with their recommendations and unwilling to make any of their suggested changes. The team gave her prescription for a pain medication at a reduced dose—not, of course, what Tara wanted.

Tara returned to the Acres and handed the nurse on duty a prescription that was visibly tampered with, that is, the physician's dosage was overwritten.

The nurse confronted her. "This looks forged, Tara. What's going on?"

"The doctor told me he wanted a higher dose. I thought I'd save some time and correct his mistake for him."

"Nice try," the nurse laughed. She then called me.

There was not much that I could do myself. I did have a talk with Maxine, however, and reminded her that alteration of any prescription was illegal.

"As the administrator, you might call the police," I said, but I had overlooked more important facts: Tara was a paying customer and had a good payer source.

"Everyone is entitled to a few mistakes," replied Maxine.

The facility census was low at the time. So what if Ms. Duran broke rule after rule, not to mention laws. The fact that she weighed on staff morale was neither here nor there. If staff were exasperated, they could be replaced.

Tara would have dropped me if she could. She made call after call to other physicians to get an appointment to transfer care. Not too shockingly, no one would take her. A drug addict on the make is easier to spot than one might think.

Stuck with me, Tara grew desperate. She began to write me lengthy notes and letters. I was cruel, misunderstanding, and vain. I cared only about my reputation. She was in the process of suing me, she warned, and was contacting the medical board.

I had little to say. I had provided good care and done nothing wrong. Yet the situation began to take its toll, draining me of time and emotional energy, and leading me to a new appreciation of those colleagues that had declined to continue to see Tara as a patient. My pride in the ability to handle anyone, any time, took a fall.

Tara was relentless. She dialed 911—for pain—and actually did get admitted to a hospital for observation overnight. Back in the facility again, she called me with the list of her demands. More pain meds. Many more. "I have a right to them," she screamed into the phone. When I refused to talk to her unless she stopped screaming, she hung up and faxed me a list of dosages and times of administration for specific narcotics.

As I was to discover, Tara was in a bind. Her trip to the hospital had actually led to a reduction in pain medications by the emergency room doctor. She needed me to make up the difference. When I refused, she went on strike, if in a self-destructive way.

She began to have seizures, which had been well controlled in the past. The levels of the thinner in her blood also become erratic. A few days later we found out why. A housekeeper came in to tidy and accidentally knocked Tara's backpack to the floor. Out fell her blood thinners and seizure medications. She had not been taking them as prescribed.

"I have the right to skip them if I want," she yelled at me. "You're the one who's wrong. You don't have the right to refuse me relief from pain, but that's what you're doing."

She continued to call; sometimes several times an hour. She was intelligent and knew that my colleagues and I covered for each other on weekends and evenings. I told them to beware.

The coup de grace came in the form of a phone call at two o'clock in the morning.

I awoke, startled, as I was not on call that day. On the other end of the line was a man who told me he was "Tara's lawyer." Unless I increased the dosage on her pain medications, he was going to sue me and ruin my reputation.

Who was the attorney who would make such a call? He turned out to be a nursing assistant at the Acres, who was dating Ms. Duran.

At a more reasonable hour that day, I called Tara to terminate my services. I gave her thirty days' notice, over the course of which time she would call me constantly with further threats and pleas. At the end of the month, however, I experienced a new sense of peace and quiet. Our relationship finally had come to an end.

Tara was the first patient I had ever fired. Could I have done better? Was my professionalism diminished by the fact that I could not keep her on as a patient? What distinguishes a professional from an amateur anyway? Some form of payment for the service or the product rendered is primarily what sets the professional apart. By agreeing to make such a payment, the client assumes that the professional possesses a certain level of skill or expertise. Aside from compensation, however, what is the difference? Is it a matter of knowledge, availability on demand, dedication, or something else altogether? Such was the line of questioning that arose out of my experience with Tara.

The Professional Volunteer

Other experiences led me to ponder the differences as well. An announcement came home from the elementary school, where Avishav, my youngest, attended the third grade to let us parents know that our services were needed at the school book sale. I signed up to serve a three-hour time slot and rearranged my day accordingly. Three hours in mid-day is no small sacrifice for a working parent, but my daughter's excitement that I would visit her classroom more than made up for the inconvenience.

I arrived where and when I was supposed to, and looked around for someone to guide me on what to do. By my side stood another parent as lost as I was. Eventually, a teacher approached and gave us each a cup filled with pencils and pens. When the children entered the classroom, we were to hand each of them a writing implement so that they could compose a "wish list" for the titles on sale. Having received our rather lame assignments, there was nothing left for us to do but stand on the side of classroom and observe the three or four women busily arranging tables and stocking them with books from several boxes. A few more parents stood apart from these activities and socialized; some carried on conversations on their cell phones.

Not only did I feel out of place but also superfluous. As I stood there awkwardly, I used my college psychology skills to make some observations. Confirming my first visual take, the parent volunteers could be categorized into three groups. The women (there were no men) that made up the first group were socially prominent members of our community. With a slightly superior attitude, they did nothing but talk among themselves, as if they were at a party, or poolside at the country club. Apparently, their presence alone was a sufficient donation to the school of their time and talent. The second group constituted the core—they were the ones that actually did the work and typically responded to every call for volunteers, apparently having nothing more pressing to do with their time. The third group was mine—a handful of parents that just wanted to be involved with their kids and help out a bit. Most of us in this third group had taken time off from our jobs, and there was nothing casual about our presence. I sensed that we were perceived by the other two groups as outsiders—maybe even as interlopers into what they saw as their territory. Perhaps we threatened their claim to be *real* volunteers.

Were there unwritten qualifications that had to be met to volunteer at the school? Was there such a thing as a professional volunteer? I already knew that there was such a thing as an amateur professional, having dealt with Esther Allen and her son, Eric.

The Amateur Physician

About eighty years old, Esther had received excellent care for many years from a recently retired physician in the community. She arrived at Mission Hill with a number of prescriptions, including several older medications that I did not frequently prescribe. Out of respect for the physician and also the resident, I made no changes in the medications. In all probability they did her no harm—nor did they do her much good. In hindsight, perhaps I should have intervened, as there were better medications available. I chose to act as I did out of compassion for an old lady, who clearly struggled to cope with the trauma of being removed from her home to live in a nursing home until the end of her days. As the old adage goes, however, I was about to learn that no good deed goes unpunished.

Among Esther's old-fashioned medications was a mild stimulant once used as an antidepressant, which had long ago become available over the counter. Mission Hill had a hard time stocking the medicine but eventually managed to do so at the behest of Esther's son, Eric, who argued that she would die without the drug. I knew that her life was not at stake, but we did our best to placate him.

A few years passed. Medicare Part D came into play. Esther's over-the-counter stimulant was not covered. Try as we might with a flurry of forms and phone calls, Esther would not be reimbursed for money she spent on the pills that she had taken for thirty years. As we waged our battle on her behalf, Esther went without the pill. During that time I examined her regularly and carefully and spoke to her about any changes that she might be experiencing in the pill's absence. From all indications, she was doing fine. For once, the care team and I concurred.

Her son, however, saw the situation differently. According to him, his mother was deteriorating without the missing medication.

He began to send money to the nursing home to buy the capsules at a local drug store. While he was at it, he accused me of incompetence. Why could I not get his mother's medicine preauthorized by Medicare? To him it seemed a rather simple task, and he was unimpressed by our many efforts to accomplish it. When Eric said that he would take matters into his own hands, I did not know whether to laugh or breathe a sigh of relief. Only later did I learn just what he meant.

Eric called the insurance company that handled his mother's supplemental prescription drug plan and posed as none other than Dr. Silber. Clearly he was better at answering the insurance company's questions than I was, not to mention the director of nursing, and Mission Hill's administrator. Eric triumphed. He got his mother's antiquated drug preauthorized. At the nurses' station he raised the preauthorization form over his head as if it were the Nobel Prize for the cure for cancer. Given all my effort and zero results, I felt ashamed. Yet what had Eric got? A medicine that was available over the counter.

I had to hand it to him. Eric definitely was an ace amateur. A new string of questions emerged: Why was the amateur better than all of the professionals? What skills distinguished the amateur from the professional? Should the overtures made to an insurance company regarding its prescription drug plan no longer be made by a medical professional, if an amateur's skills were more likely to produce a good outcome?

Only much later did the staff learn of a conversation between Esther and Eric, which may have led him to insist that his mother was in decline in the absence of her old medicine. She was overheard to say that she would much rather live with him than stay in the nursing home. Her remark was painful for him to hear, no doubt, and probably Eric felt guilty. To cope, we staff believed, he sought a way to help his mother that he could tolerate. He fixated on a medication that he convinced himself was crucial to his mother's health and so began his quest to secure it for her, despite the obstacles set up by an incompetent doctor and unreasonable bureaucrats.

Inside Basketball

If patients, families, nurses, insurance companies, and lawyers can second-guess physicians, we can turn the tables and do the same. My son Jared started middle school—the sixth grade. At the first teacher's conference—eight weeks into the school year—it was clear that he was having problems in math and other subjects. My husband and I were taken aback. The son of a respected computer scientist and a physician should not have such problems. Our eldest daughter had taken the same classes and done just fine, which made me want to blame Jared's teachers at first. On second thought, however, perhaps Jared did not study enough.

The solution started with an e-mail. My husband and I decided that we would "tell" the teachers how to help Jared. Well, luckily for Jared, for the teachers, and, most important, for our own self-respect, we obeyed our overnight rule regarding e-mails: We do not send them unless we have slept on the contents. This one was promptly deleted in the morning.

Instead, we would solve the problem ourselves. For three nights we supervised our son in what we hoped would be a marathon study session only to have each session deteriorate into a shouting match. Jared said that all of us needed a psychotherapist and took to his room. Should I have called Carol Sue?

Quickly we hired a tutor. Our home lives became a bit better, but Jared's progress was still lacking. The bottom line: No one was happy with either approach, and the outcomes—learning and good grades—were nowhere near attained. It was then that we recalled one teacher's suggestion that Jared join the school basketball team to boost his self-esteem.

It took some time for us to realize that perhaps Jared could have interests other than academic pursuits. Somehow our little bundle of joy believed that math was not needed, as he would become the first short Jewish basketball star ever. Why would he want to play basketball if he could write a novel or study medicine or physics? We, his parents—the "experts"—had already decided that, if he was not going to be a physician or a professional, he could at least strive to be a musician, a movie critic, or perhaps a sports commentator but never a professional basketball player.

Even harder for us to grasp was that the professional and the family had to work as a team. Jared did need a tutor—to receive non-judgmental and expert assistance in the learning process. At the same time, he also needed us to nurture and encourage him in the ways that only a parent can (as well as to put in the endless hours to help him with his work). Along the way, we came to acknowledge that professional advice born of training and experience, such as the insightful basketball idea, could be put to good use. In our case, it led to a happy ending. Although we hoped for a solid B in math, Jared achieved an A. Meanwhile, he also excelled on the basketball team. I must admit, I still do not understand the rules of the game.

The Professional Amateur

Yakoff Abramovitz's story also had something to teach me about the meaning of professionalism. Yakoff was eighty-nine years old when he arrived at Mission Hill after hospitalization for carbon monoxide poisoning from an outdated gas furnace at home. He had no family, I was told. Upon further inquiry, I learned his tragic story. Mr. Abramovitz used to be a rabbi in eastern Poland until the Nazis deported him to the Auschwitz death camp, along with his young wife, five young children, and extended family. At the end of this catastrophe, Yakoff was the sole survivor. He watched his wife and children shot execution style. After the war, he came to the United States. He moved to the city where I live and got a job in a small grocery store, which he eventually bought and ran for many years. Apparently, trauma had led him to lapse into chronic depression. He would not marry again. Known as an odd but kind man, he sold groceries to the poor at a reduced rate, and gave away candy to children.

By the time he arrived at Mission Hill, he was weak and tired. He had lost his English skills and could speak only Yiddish, the language he had spoken to his wife and children. Mr. Abramowitz did not do well in the facility. He had endured Auschwitz at age twenty-nine. What he could not endure with stoicism was institutionalization at eighty-nine. He wept like an infant during physical therapy in the communal treatment room but participated in no other way.

The staff decided that he was not a therapy candidate. However, the main problem was his culinary idiosyncrasies. He would eat fruit off the plate for breakfast, the decorative lettuce for lunch, and for dinner only the fried onions off the meat. Obviously, Mr. Abramovitz continued to lose weight.

Was he demented, ill, or just crazy? The care team ordered a full workup. Medical and psychiatric investigations turned up nothing. Perhaps the rabbi was just old. Hospice care might be appropriate. I wholeheartedly agreed.

A hospice aide, Batsheva, came to sit with Mr. Abramovitz for several hours each day as a companion. Born in Israel, she trained as an activities' assistant and had come to this country to study occupational therapy. She worked at the nursing home to earn a bit of income.

One day she asked to speak with me privately.

"Dr. Gilah, I am worried. When I'm with him, I try and eat my lunch, but he snatches my food. I'm afraid he'll be put away in a loony bin. You know, I was looking for his pajamas in the dresser drawer the other day, and all I found was a whole lot of dried bread. What should I do?"

We were puzzled. The last time that the rabbi lived in a communal living arrangement was during his concentration camp years. Did the therapy room remind him of that past? Is that why he cried?

Of course, his hoarding behavior was an effective coping mechanism developed during hard times—but why steal food from Sheva? We should have guessed sooner than we did. Yakoff's pious habits were not undermined by his dementia. No matter how hungry he was, the rabbi would eat only kosher food, which was indeed what Batsheva brought for lunch from home.

Once we contracted with a local kosher food market and showed him the identifying labels, Yakoff began to eat with gusto. He began to respond when the physical and occupational therapists saw him alone, outside of the usual group setting. He also saw a psychiatrist, who put him on medications for his long untreated mental illness. In time even some of his English came back. Yakoff never did make new friends, as perhaps he was unable to, but he did make acquaintances with a few men with whom he could play checkers and chess.

Yakoff lived to be ninety-four. Were these five of the best years of his life? I think so, thanks to the young amateur, Batsheva, who shared her observations with his doctor, who had not seen what she had.

The Shapes of Care

Each of the experiences that I relate here shed some light on my queries. Yet I am left with much to ponder, as to how nonprofessionals shape the conduct of long-term care, and the doctor's role within those contours. Clearly many that do not nurse or practice medicine exert what I consider undue influence on standards of practice and medical protocol. Often they have agendas that are irrelevant at best and too often are counterproductive to patient well-being. Tabitha, the billing consultant, can help physicians get paid more without increasing their knowledge or experience. Polly, the preauthorization representative, decides which medications patients will receive but has no medical background of her own to help her reach her conclusions. Pharmaceutical representatives, like Harry, are paid to sell their products, and influence what is available to physicians and patients, regardless of their effectiveness. Family members can influence caregivers, as in the case of Imogene, to act against what is medically best.

On the other hand, Wendy, the housekeeper, and Batsheva, the hospice aide, offered beneficial insights not obvious to those of us that provided the firsthand care. Those at a distance often are able to see things more clearly than those entrenched in the field. Sometimes we professionals are blinded by knowing the complexity of a patient's condition. It was simple kindness that led Batsheva to spot Yakoff's needs. It was plain common sense that led Wendy to see the true causes of Imogene's despair.

Eight
In Family Hands

Meadowview Nursing Home was housed in a nineteenth-century gothic mansion, which in its heyday was a landmark in the best part of town. In its present state, the house reminded me of the gloomy one that cartoonist Charles Addam's drew for his macabre "Addam's Family," and the neighborhood was probably the city's worst. The street on which the big old house sat was pocked with abandoned buildings. Businesses that flourished included a bail bondsman, a pawn shop, a Dollar Tree, a check-cashing outlet, and of course a 24-hour, drive-through liquor mart. Unofficial businesses were illicit and easy to imagine.

Although I often visited nursing homes at odd hours, Meadowview was never one of them. Deserted by day, the surrounding streets came alive after dark with drug dealers, prostitutes, and violent criminals, who were apt to roam until dawn.

The old house was a slumlord's reject when the Clark family—a widow and her four children—bought it in the 1960s. The family did not start out with a plan to convert the place into a nursing home. In fact they opened a boardinghouse, and yet they were ready and able to respond to near-penniless men and women that came off the streets, often from the emergency room of the nearest hospital, in need of a place to convalesce. Myrna Clark, Meadowview's matriarch, nursed her own mother on the premises until she passed away. Eventually, her daughters would do the same for her. The Clark sons worked in the kitchen and prepared meals for boarders in poor health; the Clark daughters fed and bathed them. Over time other relatives became involved, largely to manage purchasing and other operational aspects, but more than a decade passed before the Clarks hired anyone outside the family to help them run what had become their rest home.

How would state surveyors react to such an enterprise today? The Clarks used no such thing as a care plan. If residents needed tending to, they got what they needed. This type of care had nothing to do with regulations and everything to do with family.

A Patient-Friendly Model

By the time that I began to work there, ownership of Meadowview had passed from one family to another, although some of the original staff and many of the home's original ideals survived. What brought me to Meadowview was a strong desire to honor a retired physician, who had been my wisest, most generous mentor when I first began to practice medicine. This doctor also was a good friend and admirer of the Clarks, and he wanted me to help preserve their legacy now that the facility had changed hands. At his urging, I reluctantly agreed to become the medical director of the home so that I could please him even though it meant going against the advice of the other doctors in my practice. Thus I traveled into the unknown and never regretted one step of the way.

To put it mildly, however, the residents were neither typical nor desirable from a conventional standpoint. About half were young, that is, less than sixty-five years old, and most came from the streets or local homeless shelters. They had poor insurance, if any, and were beset by medical and psychiatric problems. In other words, the compensation was relatively low, and the difficulty of the cases relatively high.

Although the Clarks were gone, Meadowview remained in its way an icon—a privately owned family business in a Wal-Mart world of long-term care, where facilities, employees, and patients seem to be traded in the open market. Meadowview, by contrast, was a model of what a long-term care facility should be in every way that mattered most. In keeping with the Clark family ethos, Meadowview was homey. Everyone knew each other intimately. Staff might not always communicate effectively with each other, but they did care about what they were doing and about the people that they were there to serve.

Genuine hospitality was in the air. When I entered the building, I was made welcome—not because I was a doctor—but because staff members were proud of what they did. Despite the Spartan furnishings, a makeshift office was reserved for me in the far corner of the first floor. Behind a battered Chinese screen, an equally battered but functional desk and chair awaited my use, as did office supplies and prescription pads. On a small table, an old coffee pot stood at the ready, usually filled with fresh brew.

Such generosity embarrassed me sometimes, even as it touched me. I was not treated nearly as well in nursing homes with a far grander ambience. For my part, I always tried to bring a box of cookies or two for the staff and residents. Would one come to visit a friend's house empty-handed?

Despite the atypical residents, and the scant operating budget, the care that the staff offered was the best that could be given under the circumstances—and far better than that offered in most nursing homes. In my first years, when Meadowview was at its most dilapidated, I made an effort to overlook the dusty corridors, and peeling walls in desperate need of paint. Being a neat freak, I was sorely tempted sometimes to go in and clean some of the rooms myself. I never did so, however, for fear of offending someone, such was the good-heartedness of Meadowview staff, who wore their hearts on their sleeves, even if their hides appeared thick.

Circle of Care

The camaraderie extended to shared encouragement and advice, as well as to shared food, cigarettes, medication, and also clothes, as I discovered one morning when I climbed the stairs to Meadowview's front porch. There was Little Bob McCoy, taking the air in his wheelchair, decked out in a pink and lavender t-shirt designed to advertise Godfrey's, a fancy food and spirit establishment on the affluent side of town. Artistically done, the shirt featured a wine bottle, with a violin floating inside, and a plate of cheese and olives atop a keyboard. Godfrey's was known for its live music too. In fact, my eldest daughter had her Bat-Mitzvah party in the concert room there.

To see Little Bob wearing the shirt came as a surprise. He could not afford to frequent a place like Godfrey's and, even if he could, it would not be his idea of a good time. A trip to the local house of prostitution and a bottle of Wild Turkey from the liquor mart would be more like it.

Curious, I asked him where he got the shirt.

"In the unclaimed bin in the laundry," he said. "I'm not crazy about the colors, but I like what it says on the back."

He turned in his chair so that I could read the slogan: "I lost my naiveté at Godfrey's Gourmet."

Little Bob had a drier sense of humor than I thought. It was not the first time that I had caught myself out in a stereotype, although I still doubted that he cared a hoot for one bottle of wine over another.

How in the world had the shirt ended up in the Meadowview laundry?

Days later, it dawned on me. I had taken Vanessa Deepe, the facility's de facto administrator, to Godfrey's for her sixtieth birthday almost a year ago and had bought her the t-shirt as my gift. As a gift to herself, Vanessa had decided to diet in earnest and had slimmed down significantly—certainly enough to recycle a shirt that by now would be oceans too big for her.

She confirmed my hunch. "I love to see Little Bob wearing it," she told me with a giggle. "It reminds me what a good time we had that night, Gilah."

I do not mean to suggest that Vanessa tossed aside my gift lightly. No one at Meadowview was affluent. People who worked there tended to be frugal and careful with personal belongings, even items as modest as a novelty t-shirt. Once Vanessa slimmed down, she offered the t-shirt to Ludmila Sidorova, the director of nursing, who wore it to work one day and changed out of it into her uniform after she arrived. Roberta Cash, the day nursing supervisor, spotted the shirt on the back of a chair and admired the design.

"You're welcome to it," Ludmila told her. The shirt was a bit too short for her elongated torso.

Roberta was delighted. A few days later, however, she brought the shirt back to the facility. Her husband, Mike, a born-again police officer, forbade her to wear it. The shirt's prominent wine bottle and allusion to a loss of innocence were not to his liking. Roberta's submission to her husband was not surprising, given her personality and circumstances, although I did find her passivity frustrating. Still, she was generous and thoughtful enough to place the shirt in the unclaimed laundry bin for use by anyone else who might like to wear it.

Meadowview staff did tend to give what little extra they had to help the residents. A pizza party on Super Bowl Sunday was an annual event, traditionally paid for out of the pockets of several nurses. Somehow these nurses managed to persuade others to be as generous as they were. One year, when they ran into some financial difficulties and were hard-pressed to pay their own bills, they got the owner of the local pizzeria to sponsor the party free-of-charge. I had no qualms about lending them money myself. I was certain they would pay me back, which they quickly did.

Upstairs, Downstairs

Shortly after Myrna Clark passed away peacefully in one of the beds upstairs, her children, who had nursed her until the end, decided to sell the place and go their separate ways into retirement. The Ginsberg brothers bought the home—three orthodox Jewish entrepreneurs—all highly educated philanthropists who would build on the Clark family's legacy. As a first step, they paid homage and renamed the facility, although they had no financial incentive to do so. Meadowview became Clark House. The name never really took hold. Meadowview would always be Meadowview among the locals and the staff. The new signage and letterhead for Clark House did add to the staff's sense of disorientation, however, an unfortunate if unintended effect.

As the Ginsbergs took charge, it became clear that for all their brilliance they might be somewhat lacking in common sense and in grasping the obvious. Good publicity was all that they saw as needed to fill the beds, given the facility's excellent reputation for care.

"Why wouldn't every patient in the world want to come to Meadowview?" Saul asked.

Vanessa was blunt. "The place is a dump! There's never been money to fix things up. The neighborhood is bad. Do we complain? Not really. We do our best. We get along. But we're not crazy enough to have any big, ambitious dreams."

I sat in silence, unable to improve on what Vanessa had said. Not mincing words, she managed to coax "the boys" back down to earth, and gradually they began to settle into the respective roles each would take to manage what was one-part business acquisition and three-parts charitable venture. Joel, the eldest, would oversee the financial operations. Steve, the middle brother, would take charge of marketing, to the extent that it existed apart from fantasy. Administration of the facility fell to Saul, the youngest.

Saul would not simply replace Tom Clark, his predecessor, however. The staff was used to Vanessa as de facto administrator, ignoring the fact that, on paper, she had actually been Tom's assistant. A licensed practical nurse by training, Vanessa did not have the credentials to serve as a nursing home administrator, at least not ones that would satisfy the state. Tom, the eldest Clark son, did. In reality, however, it had been Vanessa, not Tom, who had run Meadowview day-to-day for the Clarks, who preferred to rely on her true talent for management. For years, the arrangement was a perfect example of how Meadowview could retain its individuality and yet operate within legal bounds. As Tom's successor, Saul Ginsberg was willing to uphold the status quo and accede gracefully to a role as administrator in name only. Unofficially, Vanessa would continue to run Meadowview day-to-day, at least for a time.

Whom Do You Trust?

The family style that was the legacy of Meadowview's beginnings as a mom-and-pop rest home managed to exist alongside latter-day regulations that governed long-term care facilities. A large part of Meadowview's operational style had been to prize skill in caregiving above all else. That emphasis was illustrated in the way that Vanessa handled Lillian White. A superb nurse, Lillian had good judgment and organizational skills. She dispensed medications with precision and speed. Her documentation and her orders were impeccable and revealed the pride that she took in her work.

In mid-career, however, Lillian was seen taking narcotics from her cart and slipping them into her purse. Heatedly she denied it, until Vanessa caught her out too. When the police came to arrest Lil, Vanessa stood by her side, and rumor had it that she later succeeded in getting the charges reduced after a consultation with nursing home lawyers.

Lil did time in prison and in drug rehabilitation, but she never admitted using drugs. Gossip said that she stole the pills for her boyfriend, who had a serious habit, or else she sold them to support her large family. In time her license was reinstated with some restrictions. Who would give such a nurse a second chance? Vanessa would.

That kind of trust and support can be critical to staff morale. Many nursing home workers endure very difficult personal lives, a fact in ample evidence among the staff at Meadowview. Roberta Cash was a prime example of someone who needed all the kindness and compassion that we could muster. Despite the family's strong faith, not all had gone well on the home front for a long time. Years ago, Roberta's fourteen-year-old daughter, Brandy, became pregnant and subsequently gave birth, first to Missy, and then to three more children with the same man, Rusty, whom she eventually married. Rusty was a convicted pedophile. When Missy herself turned fourteen, she too became pregnant. Her own father, Rusty, was said to be the dad. Shortly after the news spread, he was found murdered. Mike, the cop, who was husband to Roberta and grandfather to Missy, was accused and later convicted of the killing. After enduring the murder, the trial, and her husband's imprisonment, Roberta was left to help support her daughter, Brandy, and four grandchildren, Missy among them, whose child was soon to be her great-grandchild. Roberta was fifty-two at the time.

Throughout these ordeals Roberta managed to remain a good nurse, a remarkable feat. Prompt and reliable, she prided herself on upholding Christian ethics as she cared for Meadowview's residents. What made life difficult for the rest of us, however, was a certain passivity, if not fatalism, that must have been the source of what enabled her to cope. Her meekness proved to be a real deficit when the facility experienced a vacuum at the administrative and management levels. Although I was sad that Roberta had suffered so much, I did not feel that I could place unreserved faith and trust in her professional abilities as a supervisor. She was a follower, not a leader, and had not been one to direct us out of a crisis.

A Vacuum Breeds Absence

The day came when Saul asserted himself. Rather than simply tell Vanessa that he would like to take a more active part in running things, he used the impending arrival of a team of inspectors as his rationale. Vanessa, of course, had always handled such visits and had done a superb job. Despite its decrepit infrastructure, the facility managed to get a grudging pass after surveys because of the obvious good care that inhabitants received.

Now it was Vanessa's turn to accede gracefully to Saul. She did so without reservation. For some time, she had wanted to take a leave of absence to nurse her ailing mother in Florida. After she left, it took but a few care team meetings before the staff understood their situation. As one nurse put it, "Saul Ginsberg is a nice man, but he has no people skills," a comment that pretty much summed up the general point of view. Although he had a heart of gold and the best of intentions, nepotism would soon explain how he kept his job at all.

Intelligent and well-intentioned though Saul and his brothers were, it became clear that they would operate at a distance, and more as corporate figureheads than as hands-on executives. Highly opinionated and perhaps eccentric, the three brothers sometimes seemed more like the three stooges than the three sages. They tended to bicker with one another, and decision making was not their forte.

Without Vanessa, there was a vacuum where once there had been a strong, guiding hand. The staff grew absentminded. They began to behave in careless ways, brought on by preoccupation with the new and unsatisfactory management arrangement. Sadly, they became what I call an *absent care team*—one that generally is unavailable to the residents and their families and largely preoccupied with interactions among themselves instead. Embroiled in figuring out how to manage themselves, the Meadowview staff lost their formerly first-rate focus on the care of residents.

Regime Change

If nature abhors a vacuum, so does a nursing home. It was not long before someone stepped into the void. Not surprisingly, that person was Ludmila Sidorova, the director of nursing at Meadowview. There was nothing ordinary about Ludmila. With years of experience, she harbored no fear of the authorities, the way the new owners did. The state regulators were not any more important than Ludmila. She knew that her floor was well run, and her care plan was well crafted to reflect this fact.

Private and reserved in her manner, she was a striking person nonetheless, and wore heavy makeup to cover her acne-scarred face, as well as theatrical eye shadow and long, false eyelashes. She dressed a bit provocatively, too, as her tall, lean figure allowed for a runway look. She had only a bit of cleavage but was not afraid to flash it some. Around her long neck, she often wore unique and colorful African jewelry. She had a strong, seductive, and confident voice.

In short, Ludmila was smart and sexy. She was also respected and well-liked. The staff was not yet ready to accept her as their administrator, however. The shift from Tom and Vanessa to Saul and Ludmila had left almost everyone uncertain as to what to think. If Ludmila was sure of herself, most of the staff remained dazed and confused.

Among the few feeling clearheaded enough to act was a young, part-time dietician, whom Saul Ginsberg had brought on as his very first hire. Carla Sexton had a Ph.D. in nutritional science and did some teaching at the local university. Despite her advanced education, she accepted Saul's offer.

Immediately Carla proved to be an irritant. She studied patients' charts and made recommendations with such a sense of importance, you would think that she were running a small country.

Diet was the sure cure, she said, over and over, whether the ailment was anemia, heart disease, diabetes, or colon cancer.

No one was impressed. Carla was a theoretician on a staff for whom facts on the ground were what mattered. Meadowview residents were sick, in large part precisely because they had abused their bodies for years, and they were not about to change their eating habits.

"No one gives a rat's patuti," one person murmured when Carla first made her dietary pronouncements at a care team meeting.

What did surprise everyone was how quickly Carla became influential. Her calls for a dietary revolution began to interest Ludmila as she sought ways to lay claim as the newest quasi-administrator. One idea in particular caught her attention. The idea was to eliminate fresh eggs at breakfast.

A Matter of Taste

Breakfast was a big deal at Meadowview. I often picked up the aroma of bacon frying as I approached the old house in the morning. Once inside, I would spot folks like Little Bob as they tucked in to hash browns, sausage, and eggs over easy. Although I never partook, I could expect to be offered toast, thick with butter, to go with my coffee. If Carla had her way, however, such fare would become a thing of the past. She began to wage her campaign at care team meetings when all staff were present.

Raw, poached, runny-yolked, or sunny-side-up eggs should not be served, she explained, because they were a common source of food-borne illness. Inhabitants of nursing homes were at particular risk.

"Pasteurized eggs are safer," Carla said.

"Problem is, they don't taste nearly as good," one of the aides said.

"Health and safety are more important than taste," Carla insisted. "A ready-mix substitute is best."

Science was on her side. Among elderly persons in nursing homes, studies showed a number of cases of *Salmonella Enteritidis,* which caused diarrheal illness serious enough to require hospitalization. Subsequent investigations pointed to contaminated eggs as the source of reported infections.

Given her context, however, Carla was in the clouds again. Although her concerns would certainly apply to a large, modern institution with hundreds of residents, Meadowview was home to a small group of people in an old house with a modest kitchen. Concerns about egg safety could easily be allayed by reminding the few people that prepared food to pay attention to the freshness of eggs and their refrigeration. Given the unsettled atmosphere, however, the egg issue provoked resistance and dissension. A few staff sided with Carla to win favor with Ludmila. Most everyone else did not. In the escalation of tension, the folks that we were there to serve began to fade into afterthoughts.

The Ginsbergs waded into the spat. As administrator, Saul sided with his hire, Carla, but attempted a compromise. He would not issue an actual rule against the use of raw eggs, but he did ask the kitchen staff to use egg substitute for a six-week trial run to see how residents adjusted.

His two brothers railed against the prohibition. Steve said the fear of eggs was overblown. Joel made no effort to be polite. "The whole thing is just stupid," he said. When Carla objected, he shouted her down. "You want to ruin one of Meadowbrook's claims to fame—food fit for a king!"

I listened but did not engage one way or another. The dispute would die down without my assistance, just as other petty quarrels had in the past. As medical director, there was no need for me to step into the fray, or so I thought.

The egg dispute did not die down, however. Carla was not above spying on the kitchen staff, two out of three of whom were not in sympathy with her. Early one morning she caught the principal cook, Melba Wright, cracking fresh eggs into a hot skillet. Carla lodged a complaint with Saul. She also found evidence to support her prediction that the state would soon issue a new regulation to prohibit the use of raw eggs in all nursing homes, regardless of their size.

Once again, her research did not impress her opponents.

"You know, at Meadowview, we don't follow the regs," one nurse said at the care team meeting where Carla described the state's pending rule. "We just do what's right. The place is in so bad a part of town, no one looks at us. The inspectors are afraid to come in and want to leave quickly—and the actual care is great."

No one disagreed.

Yet it was not long before all hell broke loose.

Saul fired Melba Wright shortly after Carla complained.

In point of fact, Melba's use of raw eggs had no bearing on her termination. She was fired because she was late most days, and thus so was breakfast. Tired night nurses had to hustle to get food on the table.

Few believed that Melba's dismissal had nothing to do with frying raw eggs, however. Carla's dietary evangelism was the reason Melba got the sack, at least according to the pro-egg camp, which quickly got the upper hand, and soon made the rumor definitive.

The sense that an injustice had been done reached such a pitch that some staff members, who were discussing Melba's dismissal one night, grew angry enough to walk off their jobs in protest. As they marched out of the facility, they left behind their charges, unattended, if mostly asleep.

An hour into the unofficial strike, one of the residents was expecting his medications. He walked to the nursing station and found no one. A few of the other residents began the search and likewise found that they were unsupervised. One resident called the police, another dialed 911, and yet another called the local television station. It looked like Meadowview would finally get the publicity that the Ginsberg brothers wished for, if not the kind that they had in mind. Meadowview stood in danger of losing its license. Excellent care of its residents was, after all, the nursing home's one claim to competence. Anything less, and its survival as an enterprise would hang by a thread.

Hospice for the Homeless

The absence of executive function had led to an absent care team, and nearly brought down a nursing home that offered care like a loving family. It was a big mistake to let rumor run wild, and an even bigger one to walk off the job. Perhaps it was the remnants of what had been a closely knit group of people that kept Meadowview from disaster.

Technically, the staff on the night shift had not left the premises as they stood outside on the front porch. Little Bob, in fact, spotted the strikers and came out to tell them about the phone calls. By the time the police arrived, the staff were back at their posts and able to head off the television station, whose manager had called back to confirm before sending out a truck.

Near-catastrophe had an oddly calming effect in the weeks that followed. The bickering, which had gotten out of hand for reasons that even Carla could not figure out, came to an abrupt halt. Ludmila worked hard to rebuild staff camaraderie. Raw eggs were welcomed again in the kitchen and celebrated in the dining room. Residents, too, learned something from the incident. Perhaps complaints were best relayed to those who had the ability to remedy them, such as Ludmila, not the local television station. The residents might have lost their home.

The close call had sobered us up. Yet awareness of Meadowview's vulnerability remained. A television reporter did come along to survey the premises and wanted access to film "the most unusual nursing home ever." Ludmila managed to fend him off, but for how long?

As for me, the near-unraveling of Meadowview galvanized me to do something beneficial for a place that I had always loved. Yet I doubted that even the Einstein of marketing could bring more residents to Meadowview, despite the good care. What could we possibly do or say to attract new people to live here?

Brainstorming and experience from my own career led me to an answer: We would do the job that no one else wanted.

Together the Ginsbergs and I developed a business plan to expand Meadowview to include a hospice for the homeless. I knew that this service was one with potential; to pursue it was also the humane thing to do. Yet few homes were willing to take on the challenge. Instead, indigent people were left to die in acute care, homeless shelters, and on the street. The status quo did not speak well of a city that was trying to elevate its reputation. Sick people in the streets only worked against a city that hoped to become a top tourist destination.

Steve Ginsberg and I hammered out the goals of our plan. Meadowview was to provide a suitable end-of-life environment for prospective residents, who had formerly been homeless. Through training of current staff and new hires, we would ensure that Meadowview could respond to both the medical and the social needs of the homeless. We would work with existing hospice programs to identify prospective residents, and then care for them in what would be a collaborative effort.

Along the way, we identified common characteristics of those that might be candidates for a hospice for the homeless: People with no family, who were relatively young in age, who had a history of mental illness, drug and alcohol abuse, and/or a history of incarceration, and who had few accomplishments in life (e.g., job, family)—circumstances that can make dying more difficult than otherwise. Meadowview had been helping people with these characteristics since its inception.

Likewise, we identified challenges associated with these characteristics—loneliness, distrust of people (inability to accept care), pain control issues as a result of drug tolerance, inability to let go of life because not much has been accomplished, and an absence of spirituality. Again, Meadowview had been dealing with these challenges since its inception.

Much to my joy, the state approved our plan. Meadowview not only kept its nursing home license but went on to gain credibility and new patients. The crisis that we had lived through had turned out to be a pivotal one after all. Meadowview had not only survived, it had gained official recognition of its special niche in the world of nursing homes.

Family Loyalty

In many ways, life returned to normal after Meadowview took on an added role as a hospice for the homeless. With less fear and uncertainty about the future, the care team regained its former esprit de corps and functioned more like a normal than an absent team. The added workload led staff away from the temptation of bickering and instead to redouble their efforts to serve the home and its residents.

The novel paperwork associated with the new endeavor meant everyone had to learn the ropes, but Joel, Saul, and Steve had nothing to gripe about. The staff rallied and did just fine. Meadowview had been rescued and its care team members saved from the hardship of having to find jobs elsewhere. No doubt "elsewhere" would be a place where care was defined in terms of a regulation, not an emotion. Meadowview, however, continued to feel much like a family.

Building Trust

To be truly accepted as a trusted member of the family, rather than as a mere employee, had long required an initiation process. I was tried and tested many times before I entered the inner circle. As my reward, I took Vanessa Deepe out for her birthday dinner at Godfrey's, where I bought her the pink-and-lavender t-shirt.

The tests themselves tended to be memorable. Early on, when I was a young doctor and new to Meadowview, Vanessa took me aside. "I have a sick worker that needs you." I crossed the threshold into Vanessa's lair. The office was small—scarcely two individuals could fit comfortably. Tall stacks of books lined the walls, and on the desk lay piles of papers. The only dust-free spot was the area around the ashtray. Vanessa sat down and lit a cigarette. The worker I was to examine, Ron Cusher, sat in the chair opposite, sweating and febrile.

Ron was the head of maintenance and housekeeping, and a jack-of-all-trades. What I had yet to learn was that he was also Meadowview's unofficial stud. Between fixing the roof, unclogging the toilets, and ensuring that the kitchen was in order for city health inspectors, he was known for doing a quickie in the back hall closet with his latest partner (or two), usually a member of the Meadowview staff. There was never a shortage of ladies to pleasure an already middle-aged male, who was slightly overweight and only moderately attractive. Ron was everyone's best-kept secret, including Vanessa's, who was perhaps older than his mother.

I diagnosed him and treated him. For doing so, I gained a few points of trust and good will from Vanessa. If he recovered quickly, I would earn even more.

A few weeks later, Vanessa upped the ante. "There's a patient of Dr. Haskins that I need you to look at, Gilah. We have a problem. We're not sure if the patient is a male or female. You need to check."

Today, twenty years later, I would tell Vanessa to look for another medical director. At the time, however, I reluctantly took on this delicate assignment.

What was I to say?—"Hi, I'm Dr. Silber. I've come to check your genitals, to see if you're a dude or a lady"?

Instead I relied on my professionalism, kindness, and inexperience, which worked in my favor. The verdict? The person was a female, I told Vanessa, and earned more points in the way of gratitude. Later, it became clear that the hard-to-identify woman had appreciated my tactful approach. She wanted me to be her physician, not Dr. Haskins. Vanessa was impressed—extra points for me.

One day Vanessa told me how uneasy she felt, as she got ready to hire a new aide. At the time we were in desperate need of qualified workers, something I reminded her of.

"I don't want anyone coming in, shaking things up and leaving," was her reply. I think she would have preferred us to operate as if we truly were a family, like the Clarks—one not inclined to hire outsiders.

A Transforming Episode

In less than six months, Meadowview had completed the transition to its new status as a hospice and had done so with very little difficulty. In fact, the staff had poured extra energy into the effort, and the results were unprecedented. The faucets were fixed, the linen clean, the lawn mowed, and the menu updated.

At first Ron Cusher basked in the afterglow of a success to which he had contributed significantly. Then he grew bored. As Meadowview's Don Juan, he usually pursued petite women, but Ludmila herself began to look more interesting as he plodded through one day after another. Perhaps an Amazon was what he needed in his doldrums. Meadowview had undergone a change. He could change too.

Ludmila would be a challenge, of course. In Vanessa's long absence, she had gone on to handle day-to-day administrative functions in ways that Saul Ginsberg could not even dream of. As Ron's superior, she was unlikely to be a sexual pushover, the way some nurses were, eager to find out if the rumor was true that he was well endowed as a lover.

Meanwhile, Meadowview hummed along. The facility had a full census for the first time in its history. The staff sat down, looked around, and took a deep breath. The breath turned into small talk, and the small talk turned into gossip. Ron and Ludmila—an item? "He's a two-timer," said one ex-girlfriend among the nurses. "I'll kill him if he goes out with her."

Day-by-day, it became clear that Ron was indeed courting Ludmila. He came to work dressed in a suit and tie, which he promptly exchanged for overalls once on-site, but the aroma of cologne wafted down the halls after him all day. One Friday, he presented her with a large, colorful bouquet of flowers—Birds of Paradise as bright and exotic as Ludmila.

Later the staff stood and gaped as the two went off in Ron's car for dinner in a part of town far from Meadowview. On Monday, all eyes turned to Ron. He held his head low. Usually, he returned from his weekends ready to boast about his conquests. Now he was suspiciously silent.

"What happened?" one of the few older men in residence asked. "Weren't you able to perform, you lothario, you?"

"We had a great time," Ron answered, all aplomb. He ignored the man's jest, which was unusual for him. Ron generally liked to kid and boast about his sexual prowess.

Ludmila swept in the door then. "Ron is a great friend," she said and led him gently by the elbow into her office for their usual Monday morning meeting. It was back to business from then on.

From all indications, the romance had failed to bloom, and gossipmongers moved on to new topics. Only the innermost family circle would know the truth. Ludmila had agreed to date Ron in order to test him in a big way. Ludmila, you see, was Leonard. The lady was a dude—Meadowview's most closely guarded family secret.

I was reminded once more of the gauntlet Vanessa had put me through some years back. To be accepted into the inner circle at Meadowview, you had to earn the family's trust. The ordeal involved a series of trials, which involved discomfort, embarrassment, and perhaps some shame.

After his date with Ludmila, Ron had passed the test. His humiliation would keep him discreet.

By then Ludmila had made the grade as well. From the Ginsbergs on down, the staff had come to respect and accept her as Meadowview's new de facto administrator. Vanessa had finally handed in her resignation, as her mother needed continued care at home. Ludmila's final test had been to complete the transition to hospice, and she had done so with great skill.

Ludmila proved to be no pussycat, however. She ran Meadowview with a firm hand. From the bunker that was her basement office, she gave orders through the intercom system. Rarely did she personally involve herself in day-to-day tasks, but no one doubted that, at a moment's notice, she could resolve any problem with one hand tied behind her back.

That she commanded everyone's respect was probably because she was a receptive listener, and quick to respond to woe with honest sympathy and even with cash advances. Above all, she was forgiving. Most mistakes were quickly forgotten, as long as staff remained dedicated and caring. If Ludmila was a dictator, she certainly was a benevolent and enlightened one.

Drama Queen Cameo

Our intimate family melodramas aside, Meadowview continued to make strides in the world at large. Steve Ginsberg even began to operate as a bona fide marketing representative for what I will always think of as our Addam's Family mansion. He called Ludmila with a nursing home admission inquiry, which she relayed to me. The potential new resident was none other than Betsy Warner.

Did I know her?

I told Ludmila to take a chance and admit her. If anyone could please Betsy, Meadowview could, with its unusual combination of first-rate care and nonjudgmental detachment regarding staff and resident behavior alike.

By way of background, the rapprochement between the Warner family and Serenity Acres was short-lived. Betsy and her daughters were convinced that she needed more attention than the Acres' dysfunctional staff could provide. Although not fancy, Meadowview was homey and, since diversifying into a hospice facility, it had undergone some improvements. Its structural defects were no longer quite so obvious. More important, not even Mission Hill could offer more hands-on care from a small and devoted staff. Once again, the Warners were willing to try something new. Within a month, Betsy was installed in the best room in the house, one with a bay window, which overlooked a pretty, if overgrown, back garden.

Of course her physical and emotional complaints demanded an extraordinary amount of time from both nurses and ancillary staff. Just as she always had, Betsy complained of anxiety, headaches, and abdominal pain. She would ask for the nursing assistant, the nurse, and me—all at the same time. A variety of opinions would be given, and several different plans devised.

I did my best to reassure the staff, given my long familiarity with Betsy's case. They should expect this behavior to continue and to be patient but not unduly concerned. Not everyone was willing to listen and heed my advice.

Carla, for one, saw in Betsy an opportunity to resurrect her dietary crusade. Having laid low after the raw-egg fiasco, Carla sprang to life and threw herself into Betsy's care with renewed passion. Drama was of course Betsy's life blood. It was not long before she agreed to try a new and extreme diet of seaweed and tofu. Carla's best intentions concerned me. I feared that her zeal might do more harm than good.

More worrying still, I could soon see that Betsy's mood swings and barrage of complaints upset the Meadowview staff much more than they had elsewhere. Mission Hill functioned at such a high level. Staff there approached difficult patients with quiet confidence. On the other hand, chaos and apathy were part of the dysfunction at Serenity Acres. These traits, if not admirable, did at least serve to insulate the staff there from Betsy's histrionics. The goodhearted but less organized staff at Meadowview were more prone to alarm than I had expected. The facility's comparative smallness added to the strain, as did the need to serve the new admissions to hospice. As the day nursing supervisor, Roberta Cash could have made a difference, but she did not. Unable or unwilling to take the initiative, she made no effort to problem-solve or to help staff find a way to compensate and improve the situation. They were on their own.

Nurses began to bicker with Carla again, this time about Betsy's diet, and soon found that Ludmila remained Carla's staunch ally. If the situation did not improve quickly, Meadowview would go back to being an absent care team with regard to most residents other than Betsy, who would remain impossible to ignore.

Under the circumstances, I suggested that Betsy see a psychiatrist. To my surprise, she and her daughters accepted the idea. "After all, you're the professionals, aren't you," the youngest of the two said. "You know more about her state of mind than we do."

Betsy began to see a counselor regularly, who prescribed for anxiety and depression. Meadowview developed a care plan regarding her issues. Having done more for Betsy than for any other resident in Meadowbrook's history, the staff struggled to remain attentive when she did not respond to treatment and only became more difficult. What to do? Internal conflict was brewing.

Meadowview's uniquely homey side was still much in evidence. Ron hung all of Betsy's prized photos on the walls of her room, and placed her special lamp in the right position. Her bed was not the right height, and he adjusted it several times until she was satisfied. He also tried to find her a special mattress, apparently agreeing with me that Betsy reminded him of the fairy tale about the Princess and the Pea. One of the nurses brought her a candle whose aroma was said to be therapeutic, although even an unlit candle in a resident's room was against state regulations. Joel Ginsberg himself took a fancy to the former beauty who acted like a queen, and who could be a tart and witty conversationalist when she chose to be. He had started dropping by to visit her almost every day. When Betsy said that she was interested in learning more about the Jewish faith, Saul's wife took her to Shabbat services one Friday night and invited her to their home for dinner, where Betsy was given a position of honor at the table.

However, as time passed, the strain grew, especially between Ludmila and Joel. Why, he wanted to know, was it that the care team had found no way to make Betsy comfortable? She continued to complain of head pain, but its location and severity varied depending on the person that asked her. She grew withdrawn and rarely came out of her room despite encouragement by all, including Ron, who offered to escort her to the Friday night pinochle game if she would go. She ate little.

"I've seen her like this many times before," I told Joel and the rest of the staff. "She'll bounce back."

After exhausting themselves on her behalf, most of the staff were grateful for a respite and withdrew as well. They rarely went in to see Betsy except to provide personal care and administer medications. Her family came to visit several times a month.

Betsy did continue to see her counselor. One afternoon he asked to see Ludmila about what had transpired at their last meeting. "Mrs. Warner stated that she was sad," the therapist said. "I asked her if she ever considered suicide. She said that, yes, she had thought about it." Anyone who expressed a suicidal intention, no matter how questionable, had to be admitted to the psychiatric hospital for observation, the therapist reminded Ludmila. It was state policy.

Ludmila called Betsy's daughters. She did her best to downplay what had happened, but of course the women were upset. Neither one of them was able to come right over, which was unfortunate. The psychiatrist that deigned to work with Meadowview was contacted and arrangements were made. Mrs. Warner would be transported to the hospital immediately. She would go without her daughters.

At no time during the transfer process did anyone explain to Betsy where she was headed or why. In fact, as she told her daughters later, she assumed that she was on her way to see another specialist. Being sent off in an ambulance was terrifying. Something must be terribly wrong, she thought. No one asked her if suicidal thoughts were indeed on her mind, nor did anyone ask the practical questions, such as how she would go about killing herself. She could not walk, and had no access to medications or harmful weapons. When it came to Betsy, Meadowview staff had indeed grown distant, if not altogether absent.

Shortly after her brief stay on the hospital psychiatric ward, Betsy returned to Meadowview without hesitation. Of course, the staff was not perfect, and mistakes had been made, but she could forgive them. Her own family had shortcomings, too, but she still loved them anyway. Meadowview was her home for the moment, and, in fact, she had made friends there, even higher-ups like Joel. Little Bob McCoy liked to play cards with her, whenever she was feeling outgoing. He was so happy to see her return that he greeted her with a gift—his favorite t-shirt from Godfrey's.

Betsy took one look at its message and disagreed. "Oh, my dear, not you! You haven't lost your naiveté. You've still got it—in spades—thank goodness. Fresh as a daisy."

The Institution as Family

The Meadowview staff was really not a care team at all. It was a family. At times, staff fell into behavior much like that of an absent care team and exhibited many of the same traits. Usually, this absent quality took hold when Meadowview was undergoing enormous stress, as when there was uncertainty as to who was really in charge, and in making the transition to offer a new kind of service. In fact, when the staff was forced to behave like a care team, and not a family, it could only manage to become an absentminded one. Unable to make the transition to an institutional model of care, members focused on each other more than they did on the residents. This self-preoccupation fueled internal disputes, such as the one about eggs and led to actions that could have been dangerous for residents, such as the staff walkout.

Is it possible to be professional and still act like a family? Meadowview left doubts as to the answer. On the other hand, I think of the many mainstream facilities that I serve, and an opposite set of questions arises. Does the omnipotence of the care team in such facilities require that family-style cohesiveness be eliminated? Is care more likely to be professional, if it is offered with apathy and detachment? If so, then nursing home care must indeed be defined in terms of regulation, not emotion.

Nine
Minding the Head,
Mending the Heart

Long-term care involves more than attending to the body. Emotional outlook and mental health strongly influence a person's well-being, perhaps only more so when living in a nursing home. Depression, anxiety, dementia, and delirium are commonplace among those confined to long-term care. So is the emotional fallout from such perennial problems as loss of a spouse, loss of personal control and identity, and adjustment to life in an institution rather than life in one's own home.

Like everyone else, nursing home residents wish to be recognized and respected as individuals, and they share universal needs for privacy, autonomy, and dignity, as well as comfort and security, friendship, and meaningful activity. Spiritual well-being is another basic need of many if not most people.

These psychosocial issues receive attention in nursing homes but, unfortunately, never enough. Federal law requires nursing homes with more than 120 beds to employ a full-time social worker, and all skilled nursing facilities must provide some level of social services for their residents. Indeed nursing homes reportedly are primary providers of mental health services. Yet most residents do not receive the amount of help that they need. Alongside the problem of quantity lies the issue of quality. The government generally requires long-term facilities to use licensed personnel, but it has not enforced the rule in the case of social workers. The fact that there is a dearth of such licensed workers in nursing homes is probably no coincidence. Again, widespread unevenness exists in the quality of the mental health support that nursing home residents receive.

Despite these shortcomings, social workers do play a crucial role in nursing homes. Their knowledge of group processes can be essential in building broad investment in residents' well-being, and in helping all concerned parties, including family, facility (care team), and ancillary staff, to come together and make many of the decisions entailed in achieving that well-being.

Four Ways to Social Work

What makes an effective advocate for the emotional and mental health needs of nursing home residents? Just as experience has led me to identify certain characteristics that distinguish families and care teams, so too it has led me to identify social workers as four main types: *idealistic, self-referencing, clueless,* and *highly effective.* Although these different types of social workers carry out the same job, the ways in which they do so—and to what end—may vary significantly, as evident in some of their comments made at a lecture I will describe shortly.

The *idealistic social worker* believes in taking a programmed approach to the provision of mental health services in nursing homes. All would be well if only institutions would simply agree to proceed in certain ways and staff would adhere to the procedures step-by-step. Such a social worker tends to be impassive. He is disinclined to seek out new ways to solve problems.

Tonya Jefferies is someone that I would tag as an idealistic social worker. About forty, single, caring, and self-described as devoted to "Christian ethics," Tonya works at Mission Hill, where she sees her role primarily as a mediator among staff, residents, and families. Consistent with her ideals, she does her best to act on behalf of resident interests. She is also quick to help find alternative living arrangements for those she deems unsuited to Mission Hill's relatively formal and sedate atmosphere.

Tonya listens carefully to every resident's problems but makes no comment, although on occasion her opinion of what she has just heard can be read in her eyes and in the set of her smile. Instead, she reminds us that she has no power to change anything, but she does have a list of standardized options that we can choose from to address nearly every conceivable difficulty.

Behind the scenes, Tonya labors over every admission and discharge plan. In minute detail she maps out all of the potential problems that might befall each resident, and then devises an ideal plan of action on how to overcome them. To Tonya's credit, these plans are individualized. Yet they depart from the facts of each person's life to reflect high-minded principles in the best of all possible worlds. Tucked into each resident's file, they are miniature manifestos that staff are expected to act on, to the extent that we can.

Those among us who accuse Tonya of complicating our ability to problem-solve do not worry her. When our attempts fail, she does not blame anyone. What can she do if we cannot execute plans properly? She is only the mediator. Strikingly, she sees herself as a realist in pursuit of the ideal.

The *self-referencing social worker* tends to assume that everyone shares the same feelings and needs as she does. Such a social worker often is in search of mental health and emotional solace herself, and thus is less focused on finding ways to make life better for others, especially if the circumstances and outlook of her charges are quite different from her own.

Alma Owens is a good example of the self-referencing social worker. Somewhere along the line, she became an indentured servant to an entourage of needy friends and relatives, which is why she needs to work several jobs. "I've got grandchildren to support," is her constant refrain. Over time it has grown clear that Alma also has a drug habit to support. Her struggle to function helps her identify with substance-dependent residents at the homes where she serves on staff. Their plight is her plight is how she sees it, and she gives them her heart and soul when not too immersed in her own problems.

Alma has found a place in my own heart. I care about her struggles and can respect her efforts to help those whose problems she shares, especially as she is resourceful and often asks for advice. Yet I remain uneasy about the unknown extent of her involvement with illicit drugs. I also am well aware of the limited scope of her care. Residents who have no drug dependency register with her. She pays them little mind. Instead she seems on a constant lookout to find someone worse off than she is, to attempt to help.

The *clueless social worker* usually is one that pursued an undergraduate degree in social work in the belief that the field was relatively undemanding. Such an innocent generally finds himself in over his head, if he is actually hired out in the real world and must apply what he supposedly went to school to learn.

Page Hamilton is what I call a clueless social worker. She comes to work everyday but merely goes through the motions and does so grudgingly. She is there to earn a paycheck, not to engage in small talk with people whom she will never take the time to know well. Unlike Alma, Page does not seek common ground. Young and healthy, she simply does not relate on a personal level to the elderly and infirm, nor does she apply much of what she must have been taught at school to help them. In fact, she barely seems to understand the purpose of her job. Rather than address the needs of her charges, she walks around in a trance, not quite aware of what she is doing. Her ability to hang on is yet another indication of the dysfunction that prevails at Serenity Acres. Financial need makes Page reliable about showing up for work, which at the Acres is asset enough. She has served on its staff for many years.

The *highly effective social worker* understands that, to succeed in helping people, she must understand each individual case and sift through the pros and cons of any course of action. Such a social worker knows how to accommodate, compensate, and juggle competing interests to arrive at a positive outcome.

To my mind Hillary Berwald is just such an ace social worker, although she ended her career in direct patient care years ago. She had gone back to school to add an MBA to her MSW, and went on to become a marketing representative and later a nursing home administrator. By the time I met her, she was engaged in the business of business. Yet she remains one of the most compassionate people I know. Perhaps that is because she has suffered in life.

Her mother abandoned her as a three-pound baby in a hospital incubator. Luckily, a barren, middle-aged couple adopted her. Although they had good intentions, they were a bit overwhelmed by childrearing and made mistakes along the way. This upbringing left Hillary scarred and underloved. Unfortunately, the couple passed away before Hillary could reconcile her disappointment with her love for them.

Yet her pain did not make her bitter. Instead it gave her a compelling motivation to help others. For a time, she was the administrator at Apple Lane, a facility where I served as medical director. While she was there, Hillary ran the place the way a nursing home should be run. High morale and a strong sense of community were essentials, which Hillary never let slide from the top of her list of priorities. Her satisfaction surveys took into account the frequency of smiles on resident faces. She had enough energy left over to mentor some of the staff. One of them was Maude Hulse, a nurse practitioner, who had a similar gift for helping people. I grew to count Maude as a friend as well.

Despite her good and caring nature, Hillary continued to experience emotional upheavals, although they never interfered with her professionalism. She went through several divorces, and some painful problems with her four children. Some of her troubles were the result of caring too much. Others stemmed from a fear of intimacy. Still other tribulations could be chalked up to simple bad luck. It is said that all is fair in love and war. Hillary was engaged in both—she gave so much of herself to others while she fought to overcome the trauma of her past.

As for the business of business, Hillary definitely knew how to operate profitably: She filled the beds. Yet she made sure that the people in them received good care. She is living proof that business and compassion can coexist in long-term facilities.

Guardian Angel

The legal guardian is another important advocate of the nursing home resident. Unlike the social worker, however, he or she need not be professionally trained. A guardian can be a friend, a relative, or a court-ordered volunteer that makes decisions for someone mentally incapable of doing so. A guardian also has legal obligations to ensure that the incapacitated person lives in the most comfortable, least restrictive way possible, with appropriate food, clothing, social opportunities, and medical care. In making related decisions, a guardian is bound to honor to the extent possible the wishes and the longstanding values of his or her ward.

Maude Hulse went on to become a legal guardian, after many years as a licensed nurse practitioner at Apple Lane. Although she was an excellent nurse, Maude always yearned to do something else. Eventually, she successfully applied for a job as marketing representative at Apple Lane. I certainly welcomed the prospect of an honest person filling that position, not to mention a nurse. Unlike her predecessors, Maude would actually know the product that she would be selling.

Integrity and knowledgeability were not what Apple Lane needed most, however. As usual, the prime motive for marketing was to keep the facility's census up and its beds filled. To those ends Maude was soon found not aggressive enough, and it was not long before Apple Lane let her go. Despondent though she felt, Maude was not about to beat a retreat and return to being a floor nurse. She had thrived on the challenges of a new job, and her taste of increased autonomy and authority was not something she was willing to give up. After some research she decided to serve the legally incapacitated in nursing homes within our metropolitan area. The state would pay her about $400 a year for each person for whom she agreed to assume guardianship. In exchange she was required by law to visit each of her charges at least once a month and to otherwise be on call to act on their behalf in case of an emergency.

Maude does more than meet the minimum requirements. She does much, much more. Above all, she takes each of her wards seriously. From that seriousness of purpose stem all the extra touches she bestows on them. The amount of time she spends with her charges is no concern to her. What matters to Maude is that at least a bit more than their basic needs are met, and that they receive certain special things that are important to them. As their advocate, she also seeks to achieve what is in their best interests, even if those interests are not necessarily shared by the other parties involved, nor does she let her own personal preferences and values hold sway. Sometimes I see Maude as the only light in the dark. She is more devoted to her charges than many people are to their own flesh and blood.

In time Maude expanded her reach. She set up a small nonprofit organization, not only for her wards, but for other nursing home residents in need. Today she uses the funds that she raises to buy simple nonessentials, which can significantly improve quality of life—cosmetics and hair supplies, colognes and aftershave, and fresh flowers and houseplants. Although Maude has not excelled to quite the same extent as Hillary Berwald, she was lucky enough to learn a great deal from Hillary, whose mentorship helped her succeed.

As her success has grown, so has Maude's peace of mind. I am happy to see her old restlessness and dissatisfaction disappear, even as she remains down-to-earth and modest. Content at last, her satisfaction comes from a sense of having accomplished something meaningful and important that lies outside herself.

Corporate Caretaker

Amanda Baird stands in stark contrast. She, too, had been a marketing representative and had gone on to become Apple Lane's administrator some years after Hillary had left the facility. But her style was quite different from Hillary's. Infamous for her shrewd tactics, Amanda was superb at attracting residents, and always managed to retain a lengthy waiting list. Frequently people moved in only to leave a few days later, once it became clear that the facility was ill-equipped to handle their medical or psychiatric needs—inadequacies that Amanda should have made clear at the outset. No matter. Even a short-term stay was good for business. As long as a resident had insurance, the facility could count on several days of payment. If a few people complained about the inconvenience or the misleading information, no matter either. The staff would get the blame. Amanda would see to that herself, as she sympathized with the unhappy customers, the very objects of her deception. She might even terminate a nurse or two to demonstrate just how displeased she was.

In fact, it was Amanda, during her tenure as administrator, who fired Maude in her debut as a mild-mannered marketing representative. Amanda also fired me, although I was unaware of the fact at the time. How could that be?

I read about it in the local newspaper. Apple Lane, it seemed, was offering an upcoming lecture series, "Dementia: Hard Choices for Families," to be moderated by the facility's medical director, Dr. Emanuel Rose. As far as I knew, I had been Apple Lane's medical director for more than a decade, and as far as I knew, I still was.

I put down the newspaper and picked up the phone to inquire about the meaning of the newspaper ad. No one at Apple Lane returned my call. Five days later, however, I did receive a registered letter to inform me that Apple Lane no longer required my services. Why? Rumors included an affair between Dr. Rose and the director of nursing; a guarantee to Dr. Rose of a large retainer, if he kept the beds full; and a scheme whereby he would funnel patients to the facility from his office practice. There may have been some credence to all of these suspicions. None shed light, however, on whether Dr. Rose cared about the health and well-being of the actual residents of Apple Lane, or whether he had the knowledge needed to truly serve them.

Not long after my dismissal, Amanda resigned as Apple Lane's administrator to take on a big assignment. At one time she had run regional marketing for the corporation that owned Apple Lane as well as Serenity Acres. Now she would head up marketing for the entire corporation. She took up residence in another state. I heard no more about her until one day when I was visiting a patient of mine, Mary Beard.

"Dr. Silber, I have a guardian now. Her name is Amanda Baird. She's bringing me some new clothes."

Stunned, it took me a little while to absorb what had happened. It seemed that the conglomerate had begun to hire its own guardians to serve incapacitated residents. Amanda had taken off one official hat and put on another. Still, it was difficult to believe that she did not remain a strong advocate of the corporation even as she now served as legal guardian to some of its residents, more than a few of whom she once had worked so hard to attract to the facility. If there was a conflict of interest, no one seemed concerned. There was a care plan for each of her wards, after all.

Maude, meanwhile, did not need to make a care plan for her wards, as she was no longer on anyone's staff. What she had to do was a good job.

Sex in the Nursing Home

Every few months I give a lecture to a group of discharge planners or care coordinators at local hospitals about various issues involved in long-term care. Nursing home social workers often come to hear these lectures, too, as they deal with many of the same issues. Common topics are dementia, depression, and how to deal with families. A few months ago, I received such a speaking request from a colleague, who also asked me to come up with a topic. I had just arrived home after an especially crazy day and somewhat jokingly said, "How about sex in the nursing home?" My friend took me up on it.

The day of the event arrived, and I felt a tad apprehensive as I headed toward the hospital in what most would agree is our ultra-conservative city. Yet sex in the nursing home is certainly something that I have learned much about in this same locale. As soon became apparent, the topic was of sufficient interest to fill the hospital's main auditorium, largely with social workers and discharge planners from long-term care facilities. It was easy to spot the women that I described above to illustrate four ways of social work—Tonya and Page, Elvira and Hillary—who had kindly accepted my invitation and sat now out in the audience. Nervously I greeted my listeners and began by noting what many no doubt had observed: The sex drive does not disintegrate once a person crosses the threshold into a nursing home. What has been done in the privacy of one's own home will be done (or at least attempted) in the facility.

What should we professionals do? We should recognize a resident's need for sexual intimacy and for privacy and freedom of association. We need to be aware, too, that staff attitudes and behaviors toward sex among residents do make a difference and can have a strong bearing on how much privacy and freedom residents actually have. Family attitudes and behaviors make a difference, too, of course, and they are complicated by their intersection with those of staff.

My own experience in nursing homes illustrates some of the dilemmas that nursing homes face. Consider a few cases, I asked my audience—such as the elderly, long-time widow, for example, who befriended a newcomer—another elderly woman—who came to live in her facility. Their friendship deepened, and the two grew ever closer.

Eventually, a night nurse found the two of them in bed together, naked and kissing.

From all indications, both women were of sound mind and neither appeared in any way coerced into a sexual relationship. However, what the night nurse witnessed did not meet with her standards for ethical conduct within the facility. She reported the incident to her supervisor as a "resident-to-resident altercation," and took it upon herself to call the widow's daughter to relate what she had seen. Was it ethical to call the daughter, given that her mother was of sound mind? I suspected not.

Nonetheless, the nursing staff met to consider the situation and then develop a plan of care in response. One nurse was of the opinion that it was illegal for staff to permit sexual behavior among the residents. Another asked that a psychiatrist be consulted, because the behavior of the two old women clearly was abnormal.

What did people in the audience think was the correct thing to do? I invited them to offer their ideas.

Tonya Jefferies said that she would have given the widow's daughter a list of alternative facilities to move her mother into, and perhaps a list of psychotherapists, to boot. "There are several specialists in the city that could redirect these issues."

Elvira Owens would have responded with a laissez-faire approach based on her own lifestyle. "First check and see if anyone is being harmed. If not, just keep people's doors shut" was her general policy.

Hillary Berwald had a story of her own. "Something similar happened in my facility a few years back," she told us. "Both women seem much happier now. They eat better and are off their antidepressants."

As a second example, I described John and Mary Beard, brother and sister, who shared an apartment in an assisted living unit at Apple Lane, one of the city's largest facilities for the elderly and infirm. Grunting and groaning were heard from their apartment one evening. Neighbors and a few staff, who were walking through the hall at the time, could guess what was happening. The origin of the sounds was pretty obvious.

From the standpoint of staff responsibility, the proper course of action was not as straightforward as it might seem. By most standards—religious, cultural, and legal—incest is unacceptable. Yet these people were in their late seventies. Once again, they were of sound mind, and neither exhibited any sign of duress or coercion by the other.

Audience reaction to this example reflected the impracticalities involved in all but the most limited response. Whereas one social worker said that the Beards needed to be separated, another was skeptical. Where would the money come from for a second apartment? As long as the couple remained at the same facility, they would find a way to do as they pleased. Was it ethical to break up a family? When someone else suggested that the police be brought in, most everyone disagreed. The ages and mutual consent of the parties made such a move heavy-handed, if not inactionable.

No one had a "who cares?" response to this example, except me. "They were consenting adults, and no one was harmed," I said. "Can we change the habits of seventy or so years, regardless of how repugnant?"

I used the word repugnant, because sometimes the grounds for resistance may simply be aesthetic. In fact, a nurse at the facility where the Beards lived offered further insight into how staff might develop their stance on sex in the nursing home. "What's really gross is their weight," she confided. "Mary Beard weighs almost three hundred pounds. She can't reach to wash her privates, and she has a colostomy pouch."

Enough said.

My third example involved a fifty-year-old man and a twenty-something woman, who began to share rooms in the facility.

In this case, my audience of professionals was largely in agreement. Regardless of what staff might think, these two adults should be free to do as they pleased, as long as they were of sound mind and there was mutual consent. The nursing home is required to allow them privacy. It is their home, and they have the right to act as humans do.

"Perhaps we could designate an apartment or a private room for people to sign up for, who become couples once they're in residence," one woman suggested. By the fervency of her voice, I could tell that her facility would soon have such a room.

As a fourth example, I mentioned a case where a middle-aged man with multiple sclerosis began to date a certified nurse's assistant. Professional boundaries were crossed, of course, but such things happen. Eventually, the CNA resigned. In short order, she married the resident, who was able to leave the nursing home.

Most members of the audience were pleased to hear such a story, with its apparently happy ending. An objection was raised, however, by Page Hamilton, who surprised me enormously, if only because she had an opinion.

"The romance got started against all regulations," she said. "Any resident who has MS is much better off under institutional care. As for the nursing assistant who got involved with him personally, I would've fired her in a flash."

"What about a man, who at age eighty-five, asks for Viagra," I asked, "but hears Cialis is better and wants to know what do I think?" This particular gentleman was dying and actually had not much use for either. Yet he was unwilling to give up hope. I listened and respectfully gave him my very brief opinion.

One social worker in the audience said that she would discuss hospice care with the family. "I think hospice covers Viagra but not Cialis," she said.

What if the situation were the same, but the resident was fifty-three? In the latter case, the fellow had a chronic medical illness but not one that had impeded his sex life until quite recently, I explained. Residents and staff knew Larry to be a ladies' man with multiple partners, and people, who knew him from the community, privately were not disappointed to learn that his prowess had waned. He needed to be with his wife; that was their main point of view. Larry, however, begged to differ.

As his physician, I had to give him the facts, I told my audience. He could make his own decisions. If his health care plan did not pay for the drug of choice, he could pay out of pocket. He had no problem paying for cigarettes.

No one seemed to disagree.

In another case, a man in his eighties diagnosed with mild dementia began to make it a practice to walk into the rooms of women residents during the night. Some of the ladies were frightened by his sudden appearance, not to mention that he sometimes showed up stark naked. His granddaughter was an employee in the facility.

Such behavior was unacceptable, audience members agreed. Redirection and perhaps a room change were in order for this man, at the very least. Yet the problem might become a persistent one, and require the administration of medications or even a change in facility.

A man in his late seventies was caught fondling a demented resident. What to do?

Again, the audience agreed that such behavior was unacceptable. The man needed to be moved away and otherwise segregated from the demented residents as the first step. Ultimately, his transfer to an all-male unit might be the only solution.

I offered up another case. Brian, a thirty-two-year-old man with a brain injury, grabbed a nursing assistant's breasts. Shortly afterward, facility staff expressed concern about his scheduled outing to Hooters.

Understanding the natural needs of a man of this age is key, we agreed. Interestingly, audience discussion led to the consensus opinion that the outing to Hooters might actually improve the resident's impulse control and make the staff's sexual parts less tempting. In fact, it was Brian's mother that helped in this situation. Well aware that her son would need long-term care indefinitely, she understood that his needs would be best met if he was not a nuisance or a threat to his caregivers. Because she also realized that her son had sexual needs, she arranged periodic social outings for him as a release of his youthful energies.

Of course, staff always knocked on his door when it was closed.

As a final example, I offered a relatively commonplace situation: An elderly, demented woman was found masturbating in the dining room.

"Move her to her room," audience members called out.

No need for further discussion.

"The poor woman was blind already," I quipped, and ended the lecture with a few concluding remarks to solid applause.

My lecture was a hit. Part two would soon be in the making.

I took a break to answer a cluster of pages, which I had put on hold for an hour. Only one of them troubled me.

"Dr. Silber, Jacob Ashley is anxious. He needs something to calm him down for a while. He just heard that Gail passed."

Gail and Jacob. Instantly I was transported back to their drama, one that made any of the ones I had just used in my lecture look tame by comparison.

Gail and Jacob

Gail Winter came to Apple Lane when she was in her mid-fifties. By the time I met her, she had lost both legs as a consequence of vascular disease. She relied on an oxygen tank to compensate for lung disease after years of smoking, and she had a colostomy as a result of colon cancer. Medical debilities aside, she was not a pretty woman and overweight at that. Her character was questionable. A psychopathic liar, she was known by several aliases, and had long managed to evade jail time for theft and vandalism because of her ability as a smooth talker. When she finally was incarcerated, it was for criminal negligence. A careless smoker, she had burned down her own home with her grandchildren in it. Luckily, no one was badly hurt. Gail spent some time in the state penitentiary.

Despite a lifetime of poor judgment, her medical records revealed a lucid mind. Once tough and hardened, she had mellowed some by the time I met her, and her criminal drive had diminished substantially. Gail was not my favorite patient, but she paid me compliments and asked to look at photos of my children. If these overtures were made to win me over, she succeeded. I found myself bringing her little extras, like warm nightgowns in winter. She even manipulated me into buying her a pack of cigarettes once or twice— maybe more.

Jacob Eliot, on the other hand, was a homosexual who, like many unknowing fellows in the mid-1980s, came to find out that he was infected with AIDS. At the time, he thought he would last a month, or maybe as many as three, if he was lucky. Such was the lifespan of most of his friends, acquaintances, and lovers. Against all odds, Jacob lived on—for fourteen years—until my eldest daughter started high school. She was still in my belly when Jacob and I first met. Over the years that followed, he never forgot to ask after Shira, by name, even when his mind was failing.

I remember a summer day early on when I stopped in to say hello to Jacob. I had not yet donned a white coat and stood before him in a billowing blouse with a small lilac print.

He took stock of me before he spoke. "Lilacs are my favorite flowers. Purple is my favorite color. I didn't realize you were expecting."

Just like a man, I thought. I had seen him every week for the past eight months and only now, when I was about to deliver, did he notice my condition.

My husband, Abe, and Jacob were the same age. Abe was about to become a father for the third time, whereas Jacob faced a death sentence.

Jacob continued, "Aren't you afraid to touch me? What does your husband think?" Does he know about me?"

AIDS frightened people at the time. Fear of contagion was widespread, even if there was no medical basis for contagion without an exchange of bodily fluids. Careful to protect myself in any case, I rarely gave the risk factors a second thought. Jacob and I had bonded and had begun a journey together as patient and physician, as well as friends. Ours was a long friendship—much longer and smoother, if not as passionate, as the one that Gail and I had.

Jacob loved movies and the performing arts. His favorite night of the year was Oscar Night, when he threw a lavish party wherever he was, including the nursing home. Before he became ill, he had struggled financially for a long time as he tried to launch an acting career. Although he retained integrity and honesty, eventually he opted to work for an escort service, because it was a relatively easy and lucrative way to earn cash for a man as good-looking as he was. Perhaps this decision was the beginning of his end.

Unlike Gail, he did not ask much from me over the years, and, unlike Gail, he had a supportive family, who kept by his side during difficult times. He still mourned the death of his mother, who had passed about ten years prior to his terminal diagnosis. Maybe this loss in part explained his attraction to Gail.

How did their romance begin? Illness had not changed Jacob's sexual orientation, but it had changed his outlook. Young and relatively strong, he decided to make himself useful among the residents, many of whom were women, by pushing their wheelchairs to the dining room during the day, and then to their rooms to retire for the evening. Jacob's wheelchair escort service was much in demand. After several quarrels among the elderly women who fought for the privilege, one of the activity leaders offered Jacob's assistance as a prize to be won in one of the facility's afternoon games.

Once he began to push Gail in her wheelchair, however, Jacob's days as a game prize were over. She might have mellowed, but Gail still dominated when she wanted to. She spoke to Jacob as though she were a queen, and he were her servant.

"Jacob, help me into bed," she said the first night, and then, "Jacob, help me on with my nightie," the next.

Love Trumps

What bloomed between Gail and Jacob was left to flower on its own. The couple met with little interference from staff. Jokes and raised eyebrows were about the extent of the reaction until Gail applied for a legal guardian, and Maude Hulse took her on as her ward. At first I was elated. Maude, one of my best friends for many years, was reliable, caring, and honest. She would look after Gail and make sure that she got whatever she needed. This assignment was the best thing that had happened to Gail in a while—perhaps in her entire life.

Yet a problem arose almost immediately. Maude was not keen on Gail "doing the dirty deed," as she put it, with someone with AIDS. Gail had enough medical problems as it was, which was true enough. As a first step, she persuaded Gail to be tested for HIV. Relieved to find that her charge was uninfected, Maude then tried to persuade Gail to stop having sexual relations with Jacob. There was no indication that she succeeded, or if the condoms that Maude subsequently supplied her with were ever put to use. As slowly but surely Maude came to learn, being Gail's guardian had its limits. Try as she might, she could not protect Gail from her own self-destructive habits. Gail did as she pleased, just as she had done all her life.

Life settled down again until Gail appeared one day with an unexplained bruise. All was not well at Apple Lane at the time. Some new members of the night staff were rumored to engage in rough treatment—even in random abuse—of some of the residents. As one nurse said, "I've seen many evil people in my day but not so many in the same place."

Gail had nothing to say about her bruise. If she complained, she might be transferred to another unit or even to another nursing home. She did not want to leave Apple Lane, because she did not want to leave Jacob. She had been molested all her life, and a little more abuse was nothing new to her. What was new was her love of Jacob. She would not give it up without a fight.

A few weeks later, one of the day nurses spotted another large, blue bruise on Gail's hip. It was clear that Gail was in pain, severe enough to agree to a trip to the emergency room. The verdict was a hip fracture. How had it happened? Gail was a double amputee. Had she been dropped? Gail could not say.

"I'm an old, sick lady, Dr. Silber, and I don't remember what happened."

As Gail underwent surgery, the question arose as to whether she would return to Apple Tree. As her guardian, Maude weighed in with an emphatic "no."

After successful surgery, Gail took up residence at Sweet Penny Tree, where I continued to see her as a patient. By all indications within a few weeks, Gail appeared much happier than she had been for a long time. Staff at Sweet Penny Tree treated her well.

What happened to Jacob?

For a long time, he remained well enough to come visit Gail every week, which contributed in large part to the glow of happiness and well-being that we witnessed in her.

Maude knew, as we all did, that these visits were conjugal ones. Although she never approved of the relationship, Maude did come to accept its importance in the life of her charge—enough so to pay for Jacob's weekly cab-fare out of her own pocket.

Deception, Death, and Tribute

Although the move to another facility led to a happy outcome for Gail, Apple Lane had a problem. In the past, when Gail did not yet have the protection of her legal guardian, Maude, she had received some rough handling by staff. Administration smoothed over these "bad days" with chocolate and cokes to appease Gail. Now there was a bigger problem not so easily dispensed with. Gail had moved out of the facility after she had suffered an unexplained hip fracture. Apple Lane had some explaining to do to satisfy state inspectors.

As described earlier, nursing homes write their residential care plans from a temporal perspective—in real time—or else retrospectively or prospectively. The ***real time care plan*** develops in a progressive manner. As a problem arises, a plan is constructed. The ***retrospective care plan*** is constructed and written after a problem is found. The ***prospective care plan*** deals with problems and solutions before they occur, and does so in a politically correct, "proactive" way.

In Gail's case, Apple Lane had no choice but to write a retrospective plan. Flimsy evidence linked cause and effect. Gail was a non-compliant resident, already a well-documented fact. The challenge was to write a plan to support conjecture as to what had happened. Perhaps she tried to move to the bathroom on her own but could not? Rigorously twisting her body in the effort, coupled with osteoporosis due to her long years of inactivity, might well have caused a spontaneous fracture of the hip. The timing for such a supposition was good. Amanda Baird had just recently installed Emmanuel Rose as Apple Lane's new medical director. Dr. Rose was happy to document such a write-up as the coda to Gail's medical records at the facility. Neither negligence nor abuse was acknowledged as an alternate possibility.

Gail died about six months later. Perhaps the fracture was the turning point, perhaps not. Jacob died six months after she did, having survived for more than a decade longer than he had thought he would.

Sadly, I watched a videotape of Jacob's funeral service on a television set in my office at home. Although his death was relatively sudden, the funeral was a flashy one, planned long before his demise. Intercut into the Hollywood style were splices of another video, which depicted Jacob's life—milestones, personal anecdotes, and remarks from people close to him. To my surprise, I watched as Jacob spoke out from the television, seemingly directly at me: "Dr. Silber, you made a difference in my life."

Of course I was surprised and touched by this unexpected tribute on my television set. What of Jacob? Did he make a difference in his own life? Given the world in which we had known each other, I half-expected the answer to lie somewhere in his care plan. Yet I knew better. The short answer was Gail.

Hidden Job Hazards

As a geriatrician, I have not become cynical. Sometimes I wish I had. Instead, I diagnose myself as hypersensitive, as I take every tale to heart.

Consider my new patient, Ezra Hauptman. His son invited him out Sunday afternoon. The two went shopping for a few things and then to a nice restaurant for lunch. Instead of driving Ezra home, however, his son brought him to Mission Hill to begin a new life. Ezra was confident that he could continue to live alone, but his son did not think so.

On Monday I met Ezra and listened to his story. I squeezed his hand, but I had to let go. I needed to move on and visit Marjorie Williams, who told me, as she often did, about her three-year-old daughter, Melanie, who was hit by a car and died in front of her eyes, more than seventy years ago.

On Tuesday I met Tamila Tuttman, who had just entered Apple Lane after a short hospitalization for pneumonia. Her husband of sixty-five years died on the way to visit her. After I introduced myself to Tamila, examined her, and above all offered her my sincere condolences, I went on to see my old friend Ralph Martindale. As I well knew, his younger sister, Sheila, came to visit him at Apple Lane every day. They were best friends. Sheila took care of him through a divorce, his widowhood, and through his initial bout with cancer.

As soon as I entered Ralph's room, however, I could tell there was a problem. Slack and despondent in his chair by the window, he did not want me to turn on the overhead to brighten the room on what was a grey morning.

"Sheila's dead," Ralph told me, clearly in shock. He had just taken a telephone call and learned that she had died suddenly after an aneurysm burst in her aorta. How could it happen? He was supposed to pass first. He was a bit older, and a male, after all. Statistics were on his side. I sat and listened to this eighty-year-old patient of mine pour out his pain and then watched as he cried like a baby.

On Wednesday a colleague asked me to care for his aunt, who had come to Mission Hill for short-term rehabilitation after knee replacement. On Friday we found out that she had a rare form of metastatic bone cancer. Should I consult a specialist, who probably could do no more than I could?

Of course I do not register my patients' struggles and heartaches alone. Nurses and other members of the staff also observe them, and often they press me based on their own reactions. "Dr. Silber, Tamila is so sad. Ralph is nearly hysterical. State is due in. Please do something."

Is an antidepressant right for Tamila? Is a sedative appropriate for Ralph? Their miseries are, after all, part of life, and each of their reactions is normal. The decision to medicate must be made on a case-by-case basis, of course, and made with the uniqueness of each person in mind. An impending visit by state inspectors should never factor into such a decision, which is not to say that it never does.

Unraveling and Introspection

I do not respond merely as a professional, I must admit. Constant exposure to grief, no matter how ordinary and much to be expected, hits me on a personal level. Undoubtedly, this emotional response stems from my belief that a good doctor serves with the heart as well as the head. It is nearly impossible not to anticipate my own aging and demise as I manage everyone else's. With so many reminders all around me, how could I not come face to face with the fact of my own mortality? Sooner or later, I too will endure the loss of loved ones, just as my patients have.

I admit that there are times when I unravel in private. Not long ago, for example, I came downstairs, braced for a tough day, and saw the contents of my study piled against the far wall. Had Abe decided to pack up my things, because I needed to be put into a nursing home? In a panic, the question crossed my mind before I remembered that someone was coming to steam-clean our carpets later that day.

Yet my panic might well be appropriate in the future. I could develop rapid onset Alzheimer's, for example, something I have seen overcome many people. The fact that I know much about Alzheimer's would not spare me. Expertise can prevent catastrophe, if there is a cure for our ailments. Often enough, however, there is no course of action to take. At least dementia would offer the solace of oblivion, as soon I would not know that I was stricken. Poor Abe.

By then my train of thought had pulled out of the station and had begun to pick up speed. As I moved into the kitchen, I noticed with relief that Jared had remembered to take his duffel bag to school with him. Good. He had a basketball game. Then the thought arose: Would my son have a cardiac arrest during the game and die a sudden death? The school did have defibrillators, but would the use of one save him? If he escaped this possibility, would he be killed later that evening in a car accident, out having fun with his high school buddies? That is what happened to the teenage granddaughter of one of my patients.

Anxiety made me hungry. I would make some toast. Only the plastic bag, from which I pulled two slices of bread, jarred my mind like the bell on Pavlov's dog. The bag triggered the memory of another patient's granddaughter, who asphyxiated herself with a similar bag after a failed teen romance. I lost my appetite but not my runaway worries.

If my son did avoid a tragic teenage death, would he reach age forty only to pass away in his sleep of a heart attack, and leave behind not only his parents and siblings but also children and a wife? Logically speaking, our family has few cardiac risk factors but who knew what might happen?

And how about my eldest child, Shira, who had insisted on going to school that morning, even though she should have stayed home in bed. Would her sore throat turn out to be lymphoma?

To myself I would admit that I hoped not to survive long enough to witness my children's passing, but what losses would they have to bear? Would Shira watch her brother die? Would Avishav achieve her ambition to study botany in African jungles, only to die from a snake's poisonous venom there? She has no fear, you know. Perhaps some fear is good.

What of my own mother? Would she bury me after Abe watched me perish in anguish? How could he live alone?

How would my children judge my life? Would my tombstone read, "I have one more thing to do"?

As I imagined my epitaph, I took the first sip of my morning coffee. Filled with its warmth, I began to back away from the edge of my grave. As crazy as I get, I do know how to soothe myself and regain self-control. I know, too, that an overload of anxieties in my professional life naturally will spill into my personal life, especially when I am tired. I have come to accept these worry jags of mine, and am even grateful for the purge that they provide.

At the kitchen table I sat down to comfort myself by making a list of happy things to do: Make something new for dinner. Stop by Starbucks after school with the kids. Start a new scrapbook. How about a trip to the mall? We were going to Disney World for spring break. A sexy new bathing suit, or two, might give me a lift. I would love to buy Shira the cool dress we saw at that new boutique. Jared could always use sports equipment, and a cute stuffed animal was sure to put a smile on my littlest one's face. A wave of satisfaction passed over me, just to know that I could afford to buy all these things, and, yes, they would make us happy, at least for a time, as would the wine tasting party, which Abe and I would go to on Sunday. A night out on the town was just what the doctor ordered—and then it occurred to me: My happy little to-do list was a care plan of sorts, was it not? It was a plan to treat the symptoms of a work-related injury—emotional distress as a consequence of the day-to-day practice of geriatric medicine in nursing homes in a sprawling American metropolitan area.

For I had been hurt. I had wanted to do more in my profession than was really possible, and my enthusiasm had been thwarted. This subtle work-related injury had left me sad and sometimes anxious. Should I retain a lawyer and seek damages? Should I obtain more insurance to cover further injury? Did I, in fact, need a risk manager, or a life consultant?

Yes, perhaps I did, only I had no desire to live in a cocoon, or to protect myself in such elaborate ways. I disliked the idea of living under the edicts of a care plan as much as I objected to requiring my patients to do so.

As for the material satisfactions of my personal life, how did they connect to my professional life? Was affluence a just reward for maintaining a productive career and offering creative care? Or did I work so hard out of greed? Was it my appetite for a thicker slice of *dolce vita* that drove me to take on more and more responsibilities? The answer was a bit of both, I decided: I had noble instincts, but there was self-interest too.

Certainly the attitude that I took into the nursing home each day had a big influence on the kind and even the amount of care that I would offer my patients, so self-assessment was important.

Was I too empathetic? Probably.

Did I really need to internalize every heartbreaking story that I heard? I doubted it.

How could I stop? I could make an effort to at least be more discerning. Some of the tales that I heard from patients could be taken less to heart than others. Some ideas I refused to consider: For instance, I would never decline to care for someone because he or she was emotionally trying. Other options I embraced: I was a firm believer in family getaways.

Stress—and anxieties—are shared across the spectrum of those that work in long-term care facilities. We each experience meltdowns, even as we all try hard to offer ethical care. Yet each of us has her own unique manner, and even the most professional among us struggles to operate beyond his personal beliefs and values, which do not always dovetail nicely with what is in the best interest of the residents.

We caretakers naturally influence and affect each other. Conscientious and concerned staff members, such as Maude and Hillary, help the rest of us maintain a positive outlook and feel cared for as we care for others. Ambitious folks, on the other hand, such as Amanda, promote their own agendas, trigger our insecurities and neediness, and escalate our fears.

As professionals, we must humbly admit that we are only human—just like the people we serve, who tend to demand care consistent with their personal preferences, too, rather than with what will actually benefit them.

Gail Winter was a perfect example of someone who lived by her own counsel even when it was self-destructive. Her resoluteness to do so prevailed even after she sought and found a legal guardian whose sterling principles did help her live out her days far better than she might have otherwise.

Betsy Warner also comes to mind. She moves from nursing home to nursing home in search of what she wants—not so much in search of what is good for her.

Like me, Betsy must rely on her happy lists. Like her, I would, of course, rather buck the system all together—that is, the institutional setting. Just as I avoided giving birth to my children in a hospital, I would like to avoid spending my last years in a long-term care facility. Like most people, I would prefer to leave this world from home, surrounded by family at my bedside.

Ten
Pharmacy and Fantasy

My success as a public speaker made me giddy as I swung out of the local hospital parking lot. Perhaps I could start a new career on the lecture circuit—"Dr. Silber's Series on Sex Among Septuagenarians"—or something like that. I giggled before I remembered Gail's death and Jacob's sorrow, which brought me down again.

In fact, however, it did not much matter how I felt. I was due at Mountain Grove in less than ten minutes. Luckily, the facility was a short distance away from the hospital, and I would make it on time, if I bought lunch from a vending machine. In the car I munched a granola bar and gulped down a Diet Coke—not exactly the physician's lunch that one might conjure.

As always when I drove out to the complex, I was reminded of the movie *Psycho*. Mountain Grove sits high on a hill in a secluded environment, like the one in Alfred Hitchcock's film. Geographically, this summit is an anomaly, given the flatness of the plain on which our city lies, and, in fact, it is an artificial one, commissioned by a self-made man by the name of Isaac Thurmond. According to local legend, Mr. Thurmond instructed that his body be entombed at the base of a small mountain, which he went to great lengths to create, hiring an earthmoving crew to sculpt one on his grounds. To soften the starkness of the setting, he also planted a grove of trees.

The centerpiece of the facility is the nineteenth-century house. Whereas Clark House was reminiscent of the Addams Family's creaky establishment, this one is spookier on a grander scale—more like the Haunted Mansion in Walt Disney World. Nowadays the interior is carved into administrative offices and activity rooms, but splendid Old World décor remains in the way of parquet floors, marble fireplaces, crown molding and gold-leaf ceiling medallions. The quality of the mansion does not extend to the adjoining residential buildings, however, where everything is clean but of an inferior grade. The carpets are threadbare. The walls are burnt-orange, reminiscent of an economy motel. Cheap ornaments dangle from light fixtures, and nostalgic reproductions of big-eyed dogs and floral bouquets have been slapped up in the corridors. The kitsch makes me want to laugh, as well as shudder.

A few years ago, I agreed to take on the medical directorship of Mountain Grove in response to a request from Fountain Alliance, a hospital organization with which I am affiliated. I accepted the offer without hesitation, given a number of favorable factors. I had practiced medicine at Mountain Grove for about ten years and saw a steady stream of residents—mostly professionals and retired academics from the nearby university. The new job would probably lead to my seeing a few more "high-quality" patients, that is, ones with good payment plans, and the drive time was conveniently within range of other facilities that I served.

In terms of responsibilities, I would coordinate medical care in the facility and, to that end, implement related policies—no big deal, or so I thought at the time. The dual roles associated with the director's job were ones that I had experience handling, and I had proven myself competent elsewhere in juggling clinical medicine with medical management in long-term care.

It was true that I had no clear sense of the staff. Care team dynamics were hard to pick up on, given the fact that employee transience had escalated in recent years. Before Mountain Grove bid on the facility, its fate was uncertain. Good people stayed away, or went elsewhere in search of stable situations. Yet there was a core group—seven or so gay males—mainly nurses or certified nursing assistants—who had worked at Mountain Grove for many years. They seemed competent and caring, even if they did keep to themselves.

As medical director, I started to visit the facility each week, instead of each month, to attend to my new duties. The added visits only served to remind me of the old cliché about familiarity breeding contempt—in this case for me.

At the end of my first week on the job, Donna Myers stopped me in the hall. "You've got to see residents in a timely manner, doctor."

Donna was the facility's administrator at the time. Just before Mountain Grove had extended an offer to me, the corporation had hired her on an interim basis.

Her curt remark bewildered me. In fact, I saw each of my patients at least once a month—and more often, if their needs warranted, just as I did everywhere.

Before I could figure out how to respond, Donna jabbed me again. "You've got to serve all of your patients, not just a choice few."

Again, I was taken aback. I did not play favorites, as Donna implied. What was the basis for her accusation? Before I could ask, she moved off just as abruptly as she first appeared out of nowhere.

My paperwork was not up to snuff either. "Your reports are incomplete, doctor. As medical director of this facility, you need to explain why."

I tried. I never received the information that I needed to complete the reports, although I asked the director of nursing for the data a number of times. What I said made little difference. Donna barely pretended to listen.

Every time I visited Mountain Grove, Donna came to me with a new complaint or criticism, each more serious than the last. Eventually, she brought complaints from other people too.

"This week, we've heard from two families, Dr. Silber. Both of them called me to say that they're not satisfied with the level of care their loved ones are getting; one family thinks your assessment of their dad is way off target."

Plausible, I supposed. Statistically speaking, however, at least a few families of residents at the other facilities that I served would be complaining also. (They were not.)

A week later, Donna handed me a report: Among the eleven residents that I saw at the time, three had serious issues with me. What was left unstated, however, was that all three complainants came and left the facility within a week. I saw each of them exactly once.

The situation felt preposterous, with no way to improve it. What was Donna waiting for? When was she going to fire me?

Things came to a head when a ninety-five year-old patient of mine wanted to go home. I felt that she was ready. She had, however, a few more paid days left on her insurance plan. Donna "suggested" that I tell the resident that she would be released against medical advice unless she stayed until her coverage expired.

"We all have to play ball here, and we are all on the same team," Donna said to me.

That was not my experience. I did not feel like I was on the team whatsoever. Besides, a line had been crossed. My patient's best interests were not being served, which was a major problem, to my mind. There was no way that I would take Donna's "advice" and delay the poor woman's right to go home.

I asked Donna for a meeting, and she agreed. By then, I had decided that I would hand in my resignation before she fired me. Lord knows, I had ample reason. Although I cannot say that no one has ever complained about my medical care or practice style, the number of complaints I had received at Mountain Grove in just two months exceeded the total number that I had received in the past ten years from all my other facilities combined. Meanwhile, my efforts to coordinate medical policy and practice at the facility were nonstarters, given the firestorm of criticism every time I entered the facility.

When the morning arrived for my meeting with Donna, I entered the Thurmond mansion braced for a showdown but got a surprise instead. The grand salon was filled with staff. Pale balloons and streamers decorated the air. Two large cakes and a silver coffee urn stood on the long, central table. In pretty calligraphy, a sign stood on the table, too, welcoming Dr. Silber to Mountain Grove. Donna quickly came over to shake my hand and organize a receiving line, so that I could personally introduce myself to each and every member of the staff. The atmosphere was cordial, even festive. Yet I felt more than a little unnerved. Donna was masterful at knocking me off balance, and she had proved her mettle once again.

As I left Mountain Grove that morning, Glen Johnson caught up with me on the way out. One of the "gay blades," as Donna called the male nurses, Glen quietly told me that all was not as it seemed. "But it might be good if you stuck around," he said with a certain emphasis. Like Donna, he moved on before I could respond. Only he left me with the sense that I had been tipped off, even if I did not know regarding what.

Seeing Daylight

It was Mabel Felt, a newcomer like me, who was able to shed more light on the situation when we met one morning for her initial intake exam. As a new patient of mine, Mabel had few physical complaints, but she did have a "million things" to tell me about the psychiatric hospital where she had just completed a short stay. I tried to guide the conversation, to whittle down the million things, but to little avail. Sometimes it is best just to listen.

Mabel began with her early days of child rearing. She had six children. All but five arrived when she was living in a small apartment. Each time she had a child, she became ill and more depressed. After her first child, she was in the hospital for a year. After her third child, she developed agoraphobia. "I wasn't a good mother because of this illness," she said. "I couldn't take the kids to the park or movies, as most moms do." Then she had her fourth child. Afterward she developed a terrible rash that lasted a whole year.

"Why did you have so many children?" I asked.

"I'm Catholic," she said, "so I used the rhythm method of contraception, but it didn't work well, because my periods were very irregular."

Once her family doctor asked her how often she had sex—"How many times a week?"

"Well, how about three times a *night*," Mabel laughed as she recalled her answer. Her husband's sex drive declined a bit over time, she said, but "still, he was a very nervous man and used sex as a release." From her tone of voice there was no implication that his behavior annoyed her.

Mabel had experienced many losses. Ten years ago, her husband died of pancreatic cancer. Four years ago, a drunk driver hit her son when he was three blocks from his home. He died instantly, leaving behind eight children, the youngest of whom was a ten-year-old-boy.

Three years ago, Mabel developed breast cancer and had a mastec-
tomy. More recently, her thirty-year-old granddaughter passed away
after a long illness. She had been wheelchair bound after a failed suicide attempt in college.

"Maybe it was for the best," Mabel said of her granddaughter's
death. "Some people are not meant for this world."

I wondered if she felt that way about herself.

"I'm not too worldly either," she said, as if she could read my
thoughts. "I liked living in a loony bin for shriveled-up old ladies,"
and again she laughed.

It was true that she had been committed to a psychiatric ward
three or four times in the last decade. Her treatment for depression
hardly came as a surprise, after listening to her life story. Yet she had
a wonderful sense of humor.

"How do you feel this morning?" I asked.

"My arthritis is bothering me a lot," she told me. "I'd really like
a pain pill, only I hate to ask the nurse."

"Why?"

"She's busy. Whenever I ask, it always takes so much of her
time."

"What makes you think so, Mabel? I don't see why it would
take much time myself."

"Well, before I get a pill, the nurse has to write down the dosage
in two different logs. Then she has to wait for another nurse to look
at what she's written."

A sly look came into Mabel eyes. "I heard from one of the other
ladies that she always asks for two Vicodin, but usually she gets only
one."

I began to think a bit about what I was hearing.

Mabel continued, "Do you think that the second pill is 'for the
house'?"

Quite an astute question, especially coming from someone beset by so many demons. Yet the insinuation struck home with the
force of revelation, not the delusion of a psychiatric patient. Under
constant attack, I had not seen my way clear to question Donna's integrity, or that of the rest of the staff. If Glen Johnson had offered

me a glimmer of what was going on around me, Mabel let me see daylight. I took her hunch to one of my friends at Mountain Grove, who
said he would look into it.

Myers' Posse

Once the scales fell from my eyes, it did not take long to see
how and why misappropriation of prescription drugs and other illicit
activities could flourish at Mountain Grove. In effect, there was no
care team.

The ***nonexistent care team*** is the consequence of a staff whose
members constantly come and go. Some are hired by the facility from
an outside agency and may only be in the building once or twice a
month. Regular staff turnover, even among administrative staff and
nurses, is high. Communication between members of such a care
team also is nil.

No one would say that Donna was unintelligent. She has succeeded for good reason, by cultivating managers of the corporations
that own nursing homes in our area. These friends have steered her
into facilities that function with a fair amount of stability because a
core group keeps things running smoothly even if it does not rise to
the level of a care team. In other words, Donna never has to do much
other than preside, something that she excels at. Her accommodat-
ing friends in corporate slots allow her to bring along her own group
of freelance nurses. This traveling team is known as "Myers' Posse"
within our nursing home community.

Myers' Posse positively thrives on the vacuum that a nursing
home becomes when it has no functional care team. Donna arrives
with a set of allies, as well as a set of enforcers, into facilities where
most staff are too temporary to object to her way of running things.
Most important, Donna and her gang are adept at knowing how to
keep records that will satisfy state inspectors. Wisely, they never stay
anywhere for long. Donna will take nothing but interim positions,
given her marginal administrative competence, and that way she and
her pals stay ahead of trouble.

Donna and her sidekicks are not known for making friends, and
I was not interested in becoming one. On the other hand, I was not
interested in becoming their enemy either.

Unfortunately, an adversary was exactly how they saw me. As it happened, a colleague of mine had questioned the posse's level of patient care on numerous occasions. As a result, Donna had recently been asked for the first time to step down as interim administrator before she could make her usual getaway. Once Donna and her gang discovered that their critic and I served in the same medical practice, they decided to take revenge. Complaints about me were easy to manufacture, and Myers' Posse had no compunction against doing so.

Meet the Posse

It was impressive to see how three figures could wield such influence. The least combative of the trio, Alicia Sommers was the posse's Minimum Data Set nurse, ready to solve all problems with the almighty pen. Like Tabitha Jenkins, the medical billing professional that I had consulted earlier, Alicia firmly believed that she could pull care and revenue out of thin air from her prose alone. Unlike her counterpart, Zoë Wright, at Mission Hill, Alicia was neither honest nor hard working. She was, however, shrewd and skillful.

She knew that the most important parts of a care plan were its narrative and documentation, not its enactment. In charge of the gray zone—the boundary between what was supposed to happen and what actually did—Alicia could create a reality distortion field that was readily accepted with certainty.

If a care plan did not look good, Alicia changed it—on paper, that is. Did a resident's care lack complexity? It was relatively easy to add a new diagnosis or pseudo-diagnosis, such as memory impairment, gait disturbance, sleep disorder, or perhaps simply a failure to thrive. A diagnosis of depression almost always was legitimate. Alternatively, the resident's physician could be encouraged to order more laboratory testing; something else might turn up.

For all her sleight of hand, Alicia spent most of her time on the job either exercising in front of videos or fornicating with the facility's former administrator. What did Donna have to say about this behavior? Well, nothing of course. After all, the charts were in order, and Mountain Grove was highly profitable, given the good insurance plans of the residents.

Gina McCall was another key member of Myers' Posse. Obese, stupid, and lazy, she also had a big mouth. The only thing larger than her oral orifice was her behind. Although a licensed nurse practitioner, Gina's nursing skills were poor. Nonetheless, she was the nursing unit manager, and then served as the interim director of nursing in the absence of an actual DON at Mountain Grove. No one whose skills were as poor as Gina's could manage a unit of nurses, nor did Donna expect her to. Donna was not interested in quality work. She was interested in filling open positions with loyal people, who would ferret out any whisper of discontent or insubordination. Gina was simply one of her marionettes, and Donna pulled her strings. The fact that Donna's puppet never provided me with the information that I needed to complete my reports as medical director was my fault, not Gina's.

To supervise nursing on the behavioral unit, Donna chose Barb Wilson whose primary purpose seemed to be to inject fear into the staff. Quick to delegate work, Barb spent most of her time trying to figure out how to blame others for doing something wrong. Some of her reports were factual or at least based in fact. Others were just lies, fabricated when real stories were scarce, in the same way that Donna lodged false accusations against me. If an employee was not at fault in fact, Barb simply altered her job description to put her there on paper.

There was never a time that Barb was not reporting someone for doing the wrong thing, which did result in some staff firings, most of them unwarranted. Yet the point was never to penalize incompetence but to cow and intimidate those who might take initiative. Barb's reign of terror at Mountain Grove was meant to thwart the possibility that a cohesive care team might grow up and replace Myer's Posse. Eventually, Mountain Grove would hire a competent and fair-minded administrator, and create the right atmosphere in which a strong care team could develop. As long as Donna remained interim administrator, however, Mountain Grove's care team remained effectively nonexistent. Myers' Posse ruled.

At the mercy of the posse, residents—especially those on the behavioral unit, all of whom were mentally impaired in some way—

were more vulnerable than ever. What could they say or do if they were not treated well? Could abuse be hidden in the closet? Could residents be forced to stay in the facility based on inaccurate reports and records? Who would contest their treatment? Not their legal guardians, who typically were employed by Mountain Grove's corporate owners. Fortunately, nurses like Glen Johnson worked deftly to ensure the well-being of these residents. Somehow Barb knew better than to get in their way, which was not so difficult. Glen and his small band of aces certainly kept their distance from her.

Under the Posse's Thumb

It took time for me to get to know the individual members who belonged to Myers' Posse and to understand how they operated. That was not the case for personnel who worked under their thumb. Brian Burkel and Terry Nagata were two nurses as new to Mountain Grove as I was. They bore the brunt of the posse's abuse. Fortunately for Mountain Grove's residents, they were as upright as Glen Johnson, if not as adept.

Brian came to the nursing profession just a few years ago, in search of a mid-life career change. He had worked in advertising for twenty years and was burnt-out, scrambling to meet agency demands for a new image every year or so. Then his mother was diagnosed with metastatic lung cancer. He quit his job to care for her during the six months before she died. Afterward, he wanted no part of advertising. He went back to school, and had just recently begun his first job as a licensed nurse practitioner at Mountain Grove.

Brian cared. He cared a lot. He strived to do a good job and to make a real difference in people's lives. Health care, as practiced under the thumb of Myers' Posse, however, was not much different than advertising. Marketing and image took priority, as did making money. Still, Brian made up his mind to do a good job and not let the Myers' Posse bother him.

Gina screamed and yelled. Barb found fault and blamed. Alicia wrote fairy tales about patient health. Brian just plodded along as best he could.

"I figure I can still do the work that I want to do," he told me. "No one can keep me from caring for patients in the best way I know how."

He might not be able to change the system, but he could enhance the lives of the ill and infirm. To that end, he quoted the first man on the moon: "One step for man, but one giant step for mankind."

Terry Nagata was another story. An experienced and devoted nurse, she was unable to steel herself when confronted by Myers' Posse. Without a real care team to support her, she suffered, although she was not lacking in grit. As a divorced mother, she was also grandmother to the two children of her teenaged daughter, all of whom depended on her for income and a place to live. To add to her woes, Terry was diagnosed with breast cancer, shortly after she started to work at Mountain Grove. Although it was a curable form, for a time she spent many days undergoing chemotherapy.

Terry considered herself lucky to have landed a job before her diagnosis. She needed to keep it, given her high medical bills. Summoning what was left of her energy, she returned to work as soon as she could.

On the first day back, Gina reprimanded her for taking time off. Barb threatened to issue a formal complaint against her for abusing sick leave. Alicia insisted that she bring in supporting documentation from her doctor.

In tears, Terry asked me to intercede.

Donna agreed to tell her posse to back off. Her willingness to do so surprised me a little, but I was not yet aware that Mountain Grove had completed its private investigation of the facility.

Fresh New Pharmacy

Donna's stance became clear once the investigative report came out. There was a drug problem at Mountain Grove, all right. The problem began well before Myers' Posse had come to the facility. Still, thefts and double-dipping had escalated on Donna's watch. Suddenly she and her posse were under enormous pressure to acquit themselves. The seriousness of the situation required them to focus single-mindedly. Gone was the time for small pleasures, such as provoking Brian and persecuting Terry.

Donna was good at landing on her feet, of course. Her interim status gave her an advantage—corporate leniency. Her primary responsibility, after all, was simply to keep the facility afloat until a permanent administrator could be hired. For once staff transience was an institutional advantage too. She could bar the rehire of any temporary employee without cause. The hard part came when she had to terminate a member of her own posse—Gina—as interim director of nursing. Donna hated to do it but saw no choice, as Gina's termination was the express wish of the top folks at Mountain Grove.

Afterward Donna complained bitterly. She had had to fire a "perfectly good" nursing director to placate headquarters. What an injustice. Donna refused to accept Gina's part in what had happened, despite the evidence against her in the investigator's report. The real fault lay in the negligence of the pharmaceutical vendor that filled resident prescriptions, Donna maintained, which led her to make an executive decision: Mountain Grove would change vendors. In truth, the pharmacy was at no fault at all.

Under the circumstances, however, Mountain Grove welcomed any change that would distance the facility from scandal. A fresh start with a new pharmacy seemed like a good idea, and indeed our new supplier gave us cause for celebration when the facility's bill came in at almost a third less than it used to be. Residents that paid privately were happy, and so were nurses, who had fewer records to keep and fewer orders to refill, now that Gina had been let go.

Yet I began to feel uneasy. Staff made certain comments that jumped out at me.

"Tillie's blood pressure is up."

"Joe's blood sugars are sky high. Is his family bringing in cake again?"

Positive comments also gave me pause.

"Annie is much more alert—have you noticed? She's not as doped up as she used to be."

"Priscilla's a happy customer. She takes a whole lot less morning pills now."

At about this time, my home telephone rang me awake at three in the morning. Amy Knust was having a seizure. She had not had one in years. I had no reason to suspect that her prescription orders had changed, as I was the only one who could have altered them. Yet, on a hunch, I asked for the dosage of her seizure medications anyway.

"None," the nurse replied.

I have many patients, my memory is not perfect, and I had been just rousted from deep sleep, but this much I knew: Amy Knust was on several medications for seizures. Over the years I have had to watch her dosage carefully. If she had too little, she went into convulsions. If she had too much, she became confused and psychotic.

I had Amy transferred to the emergency room. Her condition was serious, but she could be treated, and she did fully recover after a short in-patient stay. The experience compelled me to look into the situation further. Amy, it turned out, was not receiving several other medications that she had been on for years.

Alarmed, I saw the need for wholesale investigation. It would take time that, under normal circumstances, I would not wish to give to a facility that had not treated me well. (Clearly, Mountain Grove was turning out to be more trouble than it was worth.) Yet I could hardly walk away. Residents could not be marooned. They needed protection.

I took the problem up with Leila Marx, the new director of nursing, whom Mountain Grove had hired on a permanent basis to replace Gina McCall. Not only was Leila cooperative, she was willing to launch an investigation of her own. "Dr. Silber, I was not here when all this was going on, but I'll get to the root of it."

Together we discovered that several other patients were not getting prescribed medications either.

How did it happen?

The new pharmacy's computer system had deleted page three of every resident's prescription orders. Residents that had only two pages of orders were unaffected. Many, however, had orders for medications that ran three, four, and five pages. In some cases, the long lists included obsolete treatments and medications, which had not been administered for some time. These variations helped explain why Mountain Grove had not noticed the glitch immediately.

Once we understood the problem, it was easy enough to fix. Yet I was left to wonder: Was reinstating the orders in full really such a good idea? Although there were some serious exceptions, many residents actually had benefited from the deletion of some of their prescription orders. It was time once again for me and my colleagues to second-guess ourselves about how and why we prescribed drugs to our patients.

Often, the first urge of a corporate entity is to protect itself against any implication of wrongdoing. Ironically, Donna, Leila, and I unanimously agreed that to do the right thing—to tell the truth—was in our best interest and that of everyone else. A mistake had been made. No one experienced lasting harm. All medications that were missing would be reevaluated for their continued need.

Corporate risk managers, however, did not agree. The solution they urged upon us was to do nothing and just change pharmacies again. If someone asked or found out what happened down the road, we had covered ourselves—we had fired the pharmacy.

Yet we were still left with many decisions to make. Were we to write clarification orders to avoid multiple medication errors? Should we discontinue some of the medications, which residents had not seemed to actually need? Did we have an obligation to report to residents and families, although no harm was done? Was the facility to report the errors to the "feds?"

Meanwhile, the pharmacy, which we were about to terminate, was eager to correct its mistake and to take responsibility. Its manager was willing to discount our bill for the next six months. Were we punishing the wrong party? Perhaps we should blame the company that had furnished the pharmacy with its computer software program.

The Koala and the Penguin

As we grappled with these questions, a melodrama unfolded on the behavioral unit. It involved Yang-gae Lee, a demented lady in her nineties, who had a long history of depression, on the one hand, and hysteria on the other. Numerous medications had been tried, to no avail. When Yang-gae had a crying jag, staff had to tough it out.

The poor woman had entered an especially agitated period at the time when Terry Nagata started to work at Mountain Grove. One day Terry brought in a stuffed koala bear and placed it on Yang-gae's lap. Ms. Lee bonded with the koala almost instantly. Suddenly she had a friend, or perhaps a child, whom she needed to nurture. She named her bear "Bo-Bae"—a Korean name, meaning "treasure," or "precious."

Terry's "cure," I believe, was borne of her own suffering—working long, physically demanding hours while being treated for breast cancer, enduring family problems, and being harassed by Myers' Posse. Her kindness left us in awe, and with another reason to question by comparison the purpose and efficacy of drugs.

Then one day Bo-Bae was lost. Staff looked everywhere, but the koala could not be found. The timing was bad. State surveyors were in the building and could hardly ignore Yang-gae's piercing cries. Should we tell the inspectors that the woman was upset because her stuffed animal had disappeared? Would that look unprofessional? The modern medicine cabinet was supposed to be our resource, not the toy box.

Reluctantly, I prescribed a sedative so that the surveyors would let us be. Then one of the aides remembered that her daughter had a stuffed penguin in her car.

"Great! Go get it."

A penguin. A koala. Same difference.

We counted on Yang-gae's dementia but were sorely disappointed. The stuffed penguin was no placebo. When the aide gently placed it in her lap, Yang-gae flung the toy across the room and roared with anger, bringing one of the surveyors to our door. One look at his raised eyebrows, and Yang-gae cried all the harder.

Of course we caretakers merely stood there, helpless fools.

A trip to the shopping mall later solved the problem. Thinking ahead, we bought two koalas and set one aside for emergency purposes. Somehow the episode reminded me of our parallel attempt to solve our administrative problems. The substitution of one pharmacy for another, and then another, did not give us what we really needed any more than our attempt to substitute the koala with a penguin. It would take much more than a change in vendors to overcome our dysfunctions as a staff.

Eleven
Who's Who and Who's Not

The personnel that stole drugs were gone from Mountain Grove. A few had even been indicted to stand trial. Yet the air of scandal lingered. As the facility's new parent company took a firm hand, corporate oversight trickled down. If Donna wanted to keep her job, she would have to ensure that staff operated ethically—or else. I was hopeful that Donna would have us all perform and excel at our duties and responsibilities. Instead, a new and more elaborate identification process was the first goal on her agenda.

Everyone was to wear an identification badge at all times. Perhaps the idea was to encourage excellence by enforcing accountability? Of course, the new director of nursing would not dream of diverting narcotics. After all, she now had her name displayed, right there on her jacket. The logic seemed undeniable.

Sarcasm notwithstanding, most people accepted the system readily enough, given how little institutional memory or custom there was left at Mountain Grove. Everyone was too busy to give it much thought in any case.

Eventually, permanent staff would be issued smart badges, Donna explained. Laminated with our names and titles, these badges would be embedded with a computer chip to operate the facility's outer doors, elevators, and parking garage. In the meantime, however, we were simply to sign in, and make badges for ourselves, along with everyone else, visitors and temporary workers alike. At each entrance to the facility, a basket soon appeared. The activities department was tasked with making each one attractive, in tune with the passing seasons and holidays. As we entered the facility, each of us was to fish into one of the baskets for a clear plastic badge into which to slide the name tags that we filled out with a pen. As we left the facility, we regulars could drop our badges into one of the baskets to use the next time we arrived.

Shortly after Donna instituted the badge system, patients on the behavioral unit grumbled that they had not been getting their usual doses of medications of late. A review of the record book for the last ten days showed complainants marked down as having "refused" their medications on some occasions. On other days, their medications were marked as having been administered.

Typically, there are always a few residents that refuse to take their medications. Sloppy records are not unusual, either. Just because medicine is marked as given does not mean that it has been received. The fact that many of the complainants suffered from dementia and other mental disorders made the situation that much more difficult to gauge and resolve. Residents were not credible, and their families were known to over-advocate on behalf of their befuddled relatives.

Yet in this case, the residents and their families protested vehemently. "We didn't refuse, and we didn't receive our meds!" They practically stomped their feet in unison.

I asked Leila Marx if she would try once again to get to the root of the problem, and she quickly did. A young agency nurse by the name of Sarah Hesse had admitted to doing an erratic job of filling the medications cart and had tried to cover up her errors in the record book. Leila and I had a talk with Sarah, who seemed truly contrite and eager to be given another chance.

"I never meant harm," Sarah told us. "I just got mixed up at first and figured it was better to skip a dose rather than double it. I know I shouldn't have fudged the records."

"No, you shouldn't have." Leila was stern. Still, she was reluctant to complain to the agency. In her estimation, Sarah was a promising young nurse in many respects.

Donna was concerned when she was informed—but not too concerned. The record book was filled out for each day and, from an inspector's point of view, looked to be in apple pie order. Who could prove otherwise?

I tended to agree that we should downplay the incident. The problem was easily corrected, and there was good reason not to broadcast another irregularity. Mountain Grove had managed to avoid a public scandal, but it remained understaffed, as news of the drug diversion spread and scared away many nurses, who were afraid of the taint.

We decided to let Sarah Hesse off with a stiff warning: One more slip-up, and she would not be welcome back.

The badge rule, meanwhile, was one that Donna continued to enforce with vigor.

Shortly after our decision to give Sarah another chance, a visitor came into the facility one Saturday evening. With a quick glance into the basket, she grabbed a badge. Impatient and preoccupied, she believed it was the one that she had created the last time she had come in to see her mother, about a week earlier. She was mistaken. The badge that Barb Wilsten pinned on to her lapel was not hers. It was the badge of Barb Wilson, the behavioral unit supervisor and member of Myers' Posse, best known for playing the blame game.

Barb Wilsten's mother, Emily, who had been diagnosed with mild dementia, still retained some lucidity and was anxious to prove it. She was among the handful of residents that had complained about medications being administered improperly over the past week. Mother and daughter were close, but Barb Wilsten had been out of town and had not been into the facility the past five days.

Who should be working on the behavioral unit that evening but Sarah Hesse, the young nurse, whose slapdash behavior was the cause of complaint. As an agency nurse, Sarah had never met Barb Wilson, who worked only on weekdays, whereas Sarah generally worked weekends. When a woman visitor neared the nurse's station, Sarah glanced at her badge and grew petrified. Sarah knew Barb Wilson's reputation for fault finding and for firing staff for transgressions far smaller than hers. In a few minutes, Sarah was supposed to begin to fill the medication cart. The prospect threw her into a panic. She hurried off the unit, ostensibly for a break but really to compose herself. After a cigarette, a candy bar, and an energy drink from the vending machine, she made several calls to her friends and family on her cell phone. At last, she had a plan. Never again would she accept an assignment at Mountain Grove. The chance of incurring Barb Wilson's wrath was as horrifying to her as it was likely. She would continue to temp elsewhere until she had enough experience to land a real job. In the meantime, however, she would summon the courage to finish her last shift with a calm dignity. Somehow.

Sarah returned to a deserted floor to continue her medications pass. Eventually, she arrived with her cart outside Emily Wilsten's room. Inside sat the same big-boned visitor, with her name tag prominently displayed: Barbara Wilson.

Sarah braced herself. Once Barb saw Sarah's name tag, she was liable to get a tongue lashing. By then, she figured, most everyone on staff must know that she was the one that had fumbled the cart last week. Barb Wilson would be one of the few that would have no problem ridiculing her openly. In fact, she would enjoy taking Sarah apart, based on everything that was said about Barb Wilson.

When Barb did begin to speak, it was to make a soft-spoken and polite remark to her mother. "Oh, here comes your medication, dear."

"I hope it's right this time," Emily answered. "Is my blue pill in the cup?"

"Yes, I see it."

Barbara Wilsten actually smiled up at Sarah, as she came into the room and handed to Emily the paper cup filled with her pills.

As Emily peered into the cup, Sarah turned away as quickly as she could, eager to move on.

Before she could exit the room, Barbara spoke again. "Sorry. I should introduce myself. I'm Emily's daughter."

As she stood up and extended her hand to Sarah, the cheap plastic badge on her lapel dropped to the floor.

As she bent down to retrieve it, she glanced at the name tag for the first time. Then she laughed in a way that sounded amazed. "Boy, have I made a big mistake," she said. "I'm impersonating the biggest fat-assed bitch I've seen in some time."

Sarah stood before her, speechless.

"Excuse me, Sarah, I'm actually Barbara *Wilsten*," she said. Once again, she extended her hand and this time Sarah took it.

"I'm sorry if my language was offensive," the woman said, "but that woman rubs me the wrong way."

Sarah had still not found a way to reply. Having undergone what felt like a near-death experience, she felt almost catatonic.

"Emily, do you need anything else?" she finally asked.

"No, I'm fine now. Just don't forget to give me my pain pill later tonight."

"Oh, I won't forget," Sarah said and turned to leave.

"Thanks, Sarah," Barbara said to her with another smile, clearly appreciative. "Thanks for taking good care of my mother."

Down the hall Sarah continued with her medication cart, far too dazed to make much more than a phantom pass.

Much later, Sarah could bring herself to tell those of us on staff her story. Emily Wilsten and her daughter had left a strong impression. Despite the intense scare, Sarah had had a life-changing experience. Most of us need encouragement and a strong sense of purpose to inspire our best performance. That evening Sarah had received hers. Long after Barb Wilson had left Mountain Grove, Sarah continued to work in the facility, eventually on a permanent basis. She had become a good nurse. I like to think it was partly a result of what happened that evening.

What's Real and What's Not

Neither a major drug bust nor pharmacy hopping had set things straight at the facility, however. Someone filed a complaint with the state. We never knew who the complainant was, but we suspected that it was an insider, as specific details were cited.

A state team was due out to investigate early on a Tuesday morning after a long weekend. Alicia Sommers was placed on high alert. As a member of Myers' Posse and in charge of resident care plans, she had embroidered the medical histories of many of the residents into something resembling fiction. Nonetheless, she arrived early to work, ready to take on the challenge of interrogation. She even skipped her usual extracurricular activities with the former administrator, as she was satiated after the holiday. Besides, the presence of inspectors was not conducive to afternoon delight.

The state investigative team asked for a few charts, seemingly at random, but all had some sort of abnormality associated with medication.

Alicia collected the requested charts. After a quick look, she made a few changes and turned the documents over to the inspectors. Unlike Sarah Hesse, the absentminded nurse, Alicia enjoyed thinking on her feet, tossing ingredients and adding spice, like a creative short-order cook.

All morning long, Donna sat by the investigators' side. Her reduced posse hovered nearby, anxious to cater to the team's every request. Barb Wilson brought coffee and doughnuts and then guided the investigators through the medical records. So what if the old and infirm needed tending, the task at hand was far more important. Records were perused, key staff were interviewed, and lunch was partaken.

In the afternoon an exit meeting took place. All was well, the state team concluded. Except for a few minor discrepancies in treatment timing, the medication books were flawless. Mountain Grove received a perfect score. The members of the survey team expressed their thanks to Donna and her posse for their hospitality. They also expressed their sympathy. Most likely, they implied, the complaint had stemmed from the actions of an employee that was poorly trained, or else disgruntled.

In fact, the state inspectors turned out to anticipate the future as well as to make insightful guesses about the past. Shortly thereafter, Barb Wilson dressed down Christine Rich, one of the few long-time employees at Mountain Grove. The bad review that Barb gave Christine was unfair and inaccurate, but what recourse did this employee have? Could she go to the administrator—the chief of the clan? Her recourse was revenge.

Christine worked in medical records and had access to files that predated the ones that Alicia Sommers had recreated to cover up the botched administration of medications on account of the pharmacy's computer glitch and Sarah Hesse's shortcomings. One evening, Christine faxed some original, unvarnished records to the state.

A reinvestigation ensued. What was real and what was not? The state wanted to know.

Donna rose to the occasion and in fact entered into her glory. Overcoming suspicion and distrust was her forte. The inspectors were treated to a special reception, where Donna entertained everyone at table with wonderfully funny stories. Her repartee had everyone in stitches.

"Sugar flowed from Donna's lips that day," Brian later said. "How could the investigative team tell that she was lying through her teeth?"

Alicia was masterful at concealing discrepancies, so that when the inspectors compared the two sets of documents side by side, each was equally credible. Which one to believe—the one supplied by the facility's administrator and her top staff—or the set hastily submitted by a lone, lower-tier employee, who had just received a poor performance review?

Donna's team won the re-inspection. Mountain Grove received no citations for improper administration of medication. Everything was fine. All the residents received their medications properly and always had. Fantasy prevailed.

Who's Real and Who's Not

Myers' Posse is an extreme example of an ordinary phenomenon. Most nursing home staffs have their cliques and their social pecking orders. The people that live there do too. In nearly every facility in which I have worked, an inner circle of residents wields influence. Remarkably, such circles are almost always made up of the same cast of characters—a "pregnant woman," a "nanny," and a "grieving woman." On occasion a man tries to join the clique, but invariably he fails.

Usually, the pregnant member of the clique has fairly advanced dementia but is highly verbal and ambulatory. She is expecting a baby and is due to go into labor at any minute. It is unwise to try and convince her otherwise. Totally content, such women glow with the radiance of a mother-to-be.

The nanny is a woman that carries around a baby doll, which she nurtures, just as Yang-gae Lee nurtured her koala.

The crying lady is just that. She cries and cries, and there is no consoling her. She is the yin to the yang of the expectant mother.

The men that occasionally take an interest in joining such a group usually are confused. Often they believe that they are on the job and that the facility is their former place of work.

For a time, Mountain Grove was without such a clique. Its resident pregnant woman passed away, and its nanny had been discharged to live with her daughter. Only the crying woman remained.

The situation changed with the admission of two new residents, Hilda Smith and Freda Schmidt, on the same evening. Freda was assigned to Room 144D (door) and Hilda to Room 144W (window). As part of the admissions process, a nurse recounted each woman's diagnoses and medications, and I listened carefully. The two had much in common. Both ladies had diabetes, hypertension, and coronary disease. Each also had recently undergone an elective hip replacement and had come to Mountain Grove for rehabilitation. Hilda and Freda were the same age—eighty-five-years old. Before long, they would become known in the facility as "the twins."

Yet there were important differences between them. Freda was on a blood thinner, Coumadin, which needed to be closely monitored, whereas Hilda did not take any medication of note. Freda also had a history of mental illness, and exhibited "walky-talky dementia" of a fairly advanced form. Mobile and highly verbal, she answered questions in ways that appeared appropriate to the uninitiated. In reality, Freda was clueless, whereas Hilda was lucid.

Without ado, Hilda and Freda were admitted, and the two settled into their shared room. When a shift change took place later that first night, Budd Jones came on duty. He had just graduated from school, and Mountain Grove was the first to employ him as a nurse. A friend of Brian Burkel's, Budd was eager to succeed, and he did everything by the book.

That evening he proceeded with his medication pass and met Freda and Hilda for the first time. When he offered Freda her Coumadin, she shook her head.

"No thanks. I'm pregnant, you see, and I don't want to hurt the baby."

In his record book, Budd noted that Freda had refused her medication. Later, however, he circled back to assess the medical records of the new resident. What Budd lacked in experience, he more than compensated for in curiosity and zeal. Freda Schmidt's records indicated that she had had a tubal ligation years ago. She was too old to have a baby, in any case, and yet he had read in the news somewhere about this sort of thing happening. He would take his patient's word for it and discuss the issue with me. There was no emergency, he calculated, unless, of course, she went into labor. Freda had just had surgery on her hip. She might dislodge something in the throes of giving birth. Budd had an uneasy night, having given himself something to worry about.

Before too long, another newcomer arrived. Overnight Helen Green became Mountain Grove's latest nanny. She wheeled through the corridors with Judith—her six-month-old daughter—a baby doll to the rest of us. When she learned that Freda Schmidt was expecting, Helen volunteered her babysitting services.

"Judith would love a friend," explained Helen.

Freda was skeptical but gracious.

In the privacy of their room, she confided to Hilda: "I'm no dummy. I see that she's taking care of a piece of plastic. There's lots of nutcakes around here, Hilda, so look out."

Unlike the others, Doris Clayborn had been living at Mountain Grove a long time. In fact she held the record for longest-term crying lady. She cried for good reason, she cried for no reason, and she cried at random. Yet Doris was not really sad. Her crying was an outward expression of neurosis. Paradoxically, her tears led to catharsis for those of us that could not cry but needed to—virtually all of us.

Sam Frankowski was the only male on the unit. He had come to live in the room across from the twins about six months before they did. A sixty-year-old attorney with early-onset Alzheimer's disease, he arrived in tow with his children, who were about to embark on a cruise around the world. Concerned about the care that he would receive at Mountain Grove, they had admitted Sam months before their departure to observe how Dad would adjust.

After a few days, the family came in to see Sam, and I joined them in his room. "I like it here," he said to his eldest daughter. "My colleagues work hard. If I roll up my sleeves, I can help make a difference."

Sam excused himself then. He needed to get back to work. "I've got a big case coming up," he said. "There are more lawsuits in this sleepy, one-horse town than you might expect." As his family filed out, their mixed emotions were palpable.

"It's all so bittersweet," one of the daughters said.

As I followed her out the door, Sam had a parting question for me. "Join me later? The Miami Dolphins are playing tonight. We could watch the game and have a couple of beers."

"I'd love to," I said. "Let me check my schedule and get back to you."

Unlike his family, we at Mountain Grove could accept Sam as he was—in the moment. We felt no sense of loss. We did no mourning for what he once had been. Sam simply delighted us, staff and residents alike. He agreed to play "Judge Judy" during our recreational activities, and he was earnest about our legal rights and options. At his request, an aide put a complaint box in the activity room, whose contents he reviewed regularly in search of actionable claims. If his advice was rarely helpful, it was always entertaining.

The cloud of mishaps under which Mountain Grove operated had still not lifted, as I discovered after I ordered some tests for each of my new patients, Hilda Smith and Freda Schmidt. When I came into the facility to review the results, I found that Hilda Schmidt was the only new admission with labs results—and who was she?

Obviously, as I could have predicted, the two admission orders got mixed up, and the identities of the two women had been melded into one. The lab results showed that Hilda Schmidt was not pregnant. Who ordered the test? Apparently, my partner on call had. He had done so to assuage poor Budd's overwhelming concern.

The women's similarities had led to the mix-up, but it was important to straighten everything out immediately. Labs were on the wrong patient, medications were switched, and names were incorrect. As I helped the nurse on duty to correct the information, Doris hovered nearby and listened to us cluck over the latest snafu.

"Hilda lost her baby?" she asked.

"There was no baby in the first place, Doris. Don't be upset," the nurse told her.

But of course Doris never really needed a cue. She began to cry, inconsolably.

The sound brought her friends out into the hall.

"I know a good malpractice lawyer," Sam said to Doris. "I'll go call him right away."

Freda, meanwhile, offered condolences to her roommate. "I didn't even know you were expecting, Hilda. Why didn't you tell me?"

"Oh, it's a long story, dear," Hilda said, smiling faintly. She was a good sport throughout the few weeks she remained at the facility for physical therapy. When she was released, she would take home quite a few stories to tell her friends.

In the meantime, she saw no need to burst the bubbles that led to contentment, and I was grateful to her. Entertaining a fantasy is often better than facing the reality—they were old people, trapped in an institution. They were losing their minds, their memories of a lifetime, and their hopes for the future.

Yet nursing homes are not supposed to surrender to such fantasies. The pharmaceutical companies certainly would not be happy if we did, nor would most administrative and corporate staff members, who value a well-run institution with as few theatrics among the residents as possible. So we have made fantasy a medical problem, even if science does not always have something better to offer. We order a psychiatrist's evaluation and prescribe anti-psychotic medications. After all, Doris cries too much, Freda is not pregnant and never will be, Sam is not a working lawyer, and Helen does not tend a newborn. Still, when we medicate residents, I wonder if we staff workers are not treating ourselves as much as anyone.

Physicians' Posse

Staff and patients form strategic bonds. Physicians do too. GeriMed—my medical practice—is an example. We are nerdy and reclusive, mostly due to the nature of the profession—who else would do such a job?—but we have been together for some time and have become a family, despite our diversity: two Muslims, two Jews, two Catholics, one Protestant, and one undecided. Politics are not discussed, but the unofficial count is three Democrats, three Republicans, one Libertarian, and one undetermined. We respect our differences, relegating certain topics to the outer limits, just as I do with my friend Carol Sue.

Yet we do socialize. I recall a holiday party where my colleagues and I discussed the instability of the environment that we work in. Changing vendors, changing sources of therapy, even changes in food services, are commonplace for greater financial gain in long-term care. Long-term care is a business, we reminded each other. So what did we expect?

We are made uneasy, too, by the other shifts and changes that take place. Diagnoses shift, as we have seen. (Depression becomes a *history* of depression to validate a care plan.) Pharmaceutical suppliers and insurance company drug plan representatives bully physicians regularly to replace one drug with another in a practice known as "therapeutic interchange." Are these changes meaningful, or are the differences between medications about the same as the ones between one stuffed animal and another, at least from the point of view of most of us? There is less incentive to confront problems like depression and loneliness head on, as long as we remain mesmerized by all the new pills to choose from the laboratories.

Dropping one physician for another happens, too, sometimes on a whim. If Freda Schmidt did not like me, she had a right to find a doctor that she did. If Sam's family wanted to pretend that Alzheimer's could be cured with a magic pill, they might fire me for my inability to provide it. Such freedom of choice raised a follow-on question—could doctors drop patients?

Could I leave Freda because I did not like her either? Could I drop Sam, because I was sick of his family's unrealistic requests—and my fear of potential litigation? Would it be possible to ask Helen to see one of my partners, because she was on too many medications that needed to be preauthorized, and I was tired of having to justify every order with the corporate office? Could I have refused to take

Hilda, because she was only going to be my patient for a few weeks of rehab, and her insurance was poor? As for Doris, well, tears make me sad.

What was the consensus of our group of GeriMed physicians when I put the question to them at our holiday cocktail hour?

Would any of us drop patients?

No, we would not.

Regardless of our individual formal belief system, we all had a solid base of ethics.

We could joke about it, however, as laughter made our stressful jobs a bit easier to take.

Patients and their families are more impatient than ever as they urge us geriatricians to perpetuate life at any cost, or else to guide them to a quick way out. In a state of restlessness, they are on the move for answers.

Moving from nursing home to nursing home is not an uncommon recourse, either, in the search for peace and contentment near the end of life. Such a change usually brings more trauma than peace, however, especially among chronic "problem" residents.

My thoughts turned again to Betsy Warner.

A Shift in Care

Clark House closed. The old family-owned rest home known as Meadowview had foundered financially after the Ginsberg brothers bought the place and renamed it in honor of the family that had created a geriatric oasis in an urban wasteland. Although civic leaders had heralded the Ginsbergs for opening a hospice for the homeless, the nursing home struggled to stay afloat. Two years after they took possession, the Ginsbergs did a benefit-cost analysis and decided to write the place off. Every resident was homeless then, Betsy Warner among them. She needed to find a new place to live.

Mountain Grove's marketing campaign to attract these residents was among the most aggressive—and successful. Betsy and her family were persuaded that Mountain Grove was the place to be.

This fourth move took a heavier toll on Betsy than the previous three had. This time the decision to move was not hers but someone else's. She did not feel in control of her destiny, something that was important to her. Shortly after she settled into her new room in a new facility, her old mood swings began again in earnest. Compassionate nurses remained in short supply. Mrs. Warner's high maintenance was met with resentment and impatience. It was not long before an agency nurse called the doctor on call one weekend and demanded a "nerve" pill for "the screechy lady." The doctor gave an order for a low-dose medication.

Given Mountain Grove's remarkably unlucky streak with pharmaceuticals, it will probably come as no surprise to learn that the dosage filled by the pharmacy turned out to be high rather than low. Mrs. Warner became confused and began to wander the halls. The nurse that had ordered the sedative tried to coax her back to her room, but Betsy only grew more agitated, and she began to fight back. When the nurse persisted, Betsy slapped her. Before she knew it, Mrs. Warner was heading for the psychiatric ward of a local hospital, where she spent the weekend. Her prior record did not help matters.

On Monday, I quickly determined that the weekend medication and the high dosage prescribed were at the source of Betsy's agitation. Fortunately, the hospital's psychiatrist had reached the same conclusion, despite her prior record, dating to her passing mention of suicide at Clark House. By then Betsy had returned to her former self—moody and demanding but perfectly sane. Shortly after she returned to Mountain Grove, however, I was asked to resign as medical director.

"There's nothing wrong with your performance," the new administrator reassured me. It was just that Mountain Grove had finally replaced Donna, and the new administrator was eager to find a medical director that could increase the facility's census. As I prepared to make my exit, I said good-bye to my patients at Mountain Grove, for indeed I would be passing them off to my successor. Betsy Warner and I had a tear-filled farewell. We had known each other for years. I would miss her. She would miss me.

I tried to reassure her, but Betsy took the changes in her care hard. Her new doctor turned out to be far better at marketing the facility than he was at holding an elderly diva's hand at bedside. Yet he was certainly thorough from a medical point of view. He reassessed

Mrs. Warner from head to toe. He studied her records. He ordered a multitude of tests, many of them duplicates, which led to a whole new regimen of medications. Mrs. Warner's spirits did not improve, however. She took to her bed. She summoned her family. She stated that she was going to die. The family sat vigil, but Betsy did not pass on. Perhaps a change of scenery was what was needed? Once again, the Warners began to look for a new nursing home.

Twelve
To Live and Die, Free and Real

I remember the first time that I went out to Forest Glen—the sixty-mile drive through suburbs that gave way to countryside, and then the series of wrong turns in the town proper, which led me to stop at an auto body shop to ask for directions to the facility. In retrospect, I am amazed that I had so much trouble finding my way. How could I get lost in a place that had just two main streets?

No one was on hand to greet me when I entered the Forest Glen Nursing Home, named after the little town in which it sat. I glanced at my watch. Despite wandering off course, I was only five minutes late. Just as I was about to walk down one of the empty corridors in search of someone to talk to, a woman in high heels and a pink smock approached.

"May I help you?" she asked.

"I hope so. I'm Gilah Silber, and I'm here to see Erin Caulfield."

The woman looked at me with mild surprise. "I'll go see if I can find her." As she moseyed down the corridor, I listened to her heels click at an unhurried pace. It was not a sound often heard in a nursing facility, at least not among staff, who tend to favor rubber-soled footwear. Another ten minutes passed before Erin appeared. Even at forty-something, Erin was a striking woman, tall and slender, with dark, luminous eyes. Also striking was the tiny silver stud in her nose.

"So here you are," she called out, and flashed a smile that struck me as wry, as if I had been up to some mischief. "I was expecting you last week," she said.

Last week? Deeply embarrassed, I was also confused. I am meticulous when it comes to making and keeping appointments, and I felt certain that I had not made a mistake. Erin did not seem the least bit concerned, however, and proceeded to give me a tour of the nursing home whose residents I had been hired to care for. Whatever she had been doing before I arrived apparently could wait. As we walked through the facility, I apologized several times for the mix-up, but my regrets did not seem to register.

"Oh, don't worry about it," Erin said. She sounded slightly bored, as if it mattered not a whit if I started seeing patients a week late.

But it mattered to me. In fact, it mattered a lot. After I returned home, the first thing I did was to verify that, yes, the fourteenth—not the seventh—was the date marked in my planner as the first day on the job in Forest Glen. If the facility staff had been expecting me the previous week, why had they not telephoned after my no-show? Instead, the director of nursing had met me a week later with perfect equanimity—or was it indifference?

Both—or so it seemed to me.

Erin's poised nonchalance was a classic sign of what I call a *passive care team*. The members of such teams can be elusive and often less available than the staff on other types of care teams. Passive teams also tend to interact less directly with patients and their families, and staff can seem remote and detached, even if they actually care.

Passive teams are anything but straightforward. Often I have found their members to be difficult to contact but irate and abusive if they find out that they were not informed about a particular matter. Occasionally they will lavish attention on a few favored residents and ignore others. Typically, such a team is composed of a core group that has worked at the facility for a long time, as well as several satellite groups that stay for only a short time. The passivity that I observed at Forest Glen, however, had more to do with geographic isolation and the pace and culture of rural life than anything else.

Slow Down and Dream

The route to Forest Glen was not a particularly scenic one. Along the way I passed a few churches interspersed with neat farms and several trailer parks, some occupied and some merely relics of another era. Every ten miles or so, a larger grocery appeared and every twenty miles, a Wal-Mart. At the center of each small town were a few local businesses and, of course, a McDonalds. One of these days, I told myself, I would find a shortcut and shave significant time off my commute. Somehow I never got around to it.

Six months later I was feeling particularly impatient as I headed out to Forest Glen on a Friday, always a busy day, especially this one, when I was getting ready to go on vacation. Five minutes into the drive, I realized that I had forgotten my cell phone (something I almost never do, as it has become almost a bodily appendage). I had to go back home and start over, which cost me another ten minutes. Once I hit the interstate, I hoped to make up for lost time, especially as I would have to inch along a two-lane country road to travel the last thirty miles to the facility. Before I knew it, a state trooper pulled me over for driving sixty-six miles per hour in a fifty-five mile per hour zone. As he made out the ticket, I lost another ten minutes, along with ninety-four dollars and some pride.

I learned something that day. The commute to and from Forest Glen was not to be rushed—it was to be enjoyed. Of course, it took some adjustment to appreciate my automotive "time out." Once I did, however, the trip was no longer a chore. Although time was ticking away—as were potential billable hours—I felt free. No one seemed to need me when I was coming or going to Forest Glen. Of course this impression was not really accurate, yet it was true that ever-pressing business and nagging household tasks could not be attended to as I traveled far outside my usual orbit.

Eventually I realized that a leisurely pace was one that some people might prefer all the time. Down a hallway one day at Forest Glen, I came upon Edith Holloway and her nursing assistant. The two were moving toward the shower room at glacial speed. At first I felt aggravated to have to slow down to accommodate them, but then I asked myself—was slow bad? Did Mrs. Holloway need to rush to take a bath? Did she have anything better to do?

Similarly, with nothing better to do than drive, I let my mind roam. Nostalgically, I recalled long rides on the very same interstate with my family, both in the remote past and en route to and from more recent vacations. Invariably, the stop-and-go of these journeys was associated with body parts and functions—which part and what function depended on the age of my three children. On the way to Forest Glen, I also recalled snippets of certain conversations with patients over the years, such as the disjointed but cathartic talks I

had had with Martin Scanlon at Serenity Acres. Martin had been dying, yet his insight grew ever more acute as he told me the tale of a
feather. I also had time to listen to music, a rarity except when I was
with my children, who commandeered the car's DVD player to satisfy their own tastes. Alone on the road, I could listen to whatever
I liked. Lynyrd Skynyrd's "Free Bird," with a run time of more than
eight minutes, is probably one of the longest songs in rock and roll
history. Soon I discovered that I could listen to the song eight times
during the drive from my home to the nursing home. For me, both
the song's words and music caught that old restlessness of mine, that
desire for new experience, which had led me to agree to serve in an
outpost like Forest Glen.

"Free Bird" wove its way into the passing scenery and my sense
of escape—and yet the song also led to thoughts of my own death,
which at first I dismissed as just another hazard of my profession in
which memento moris are a constant. Later, I hit on the more likely
reason. "Free Bird" was one of three songs that I had asked Abe to
play at my funeral. That request was made a long time ago, when Abe
and I were newlyweds embarked on a cross-country drive. Dying
was just one of the many things we discussed on our first big road
trip, along with how to buy exotic furniture, cope with in-laws, find
a cheap vegetarian restaurant for dinner, and generally figure out
how to fulfill all our dreams. We were very young, and neither of us
had the slightest sense of mortality. My request to have "Free Bird"
played at my funeral was just a random way to say how much I liked it.
Of course, my vision of the future changed over time. Yet, because of
some idle chatter in my youth, one of my favorite songs had become
an invariable reminder that my life would end. As I tell my teenaged
daughter, Shira, "Think before you speak!" But she will have to learn
on her own.

Care in the Country

Forest Glen presented other challenges besides the long commute. The staff included no male nurses or aides, and no African
Americans or Latinos either. In the city, male nurses served at most
facilities, and minorities might make up to 70 percent of the staff. By
contrast, most of the physicians that served at Forest Glen were mid-

dle-aged white men, who enjoyed barking orders. They would scream when things were not going their way.

How well would I fit in?

Very well, as it happened.

Within a short period of time, a solid bond had formed between a socially liberal, Jewish physician from a big city and a team of quite conservative, Christian nurses in America's Heartland. Perhaps it was our contrasting styles that sparked a new energy in the way that we operated day-to-day. The passivity, which I had sensed in the Forest Glen care team when I first arrived, apparently was more style than substance. We developed into a very capable team. Key to our success was the respectful hearing that we gave to each other's opinions, and our unspoken agreement not to sweat the small stuff as we strived to work together. (Like most of the staff, I even came to regard as small stuff the histrionics of some of my fellow physicians.)

We were there to do our jobs to the best of our ability. Having done so, we did indulge our curiosity about our differences. I was fascinated to hear fresh stories about lives led in what, to me, was an alien world. For their part, the nursing staff was quite interested in city life. They often commented on my clothes, and they asked how nursing homes operated in an urban environment.

What was different about Forest Glen, as compared with the nursing homes that I served in the city? The main difference, I would venture, was a greater accountability, borne of the small scope of such a rural world. Your very existence was under the microscope of a small town—you lived there and you worked there. Many of your colleagues were family and friends, so that the professional and the personal blurred beyond recognition. Jobs for nurses and health care professionals were sparse in Forest Glen. The town had one hospital, one long-term care facility, and only a few physicians in private practice. A job close to home was cherished. The next town was twenty miles away. The one after that was fifty—a long drive in a storm, or when your child was ill, and you needed to rush home unexpectedly. The bottom line? You would not risk the poor performance or absenteeism that would lead to your being fired—because you could not simply find another job in the nursing home across the street—a common practice in the city.

Weekend staffing levels were thus another distinction. Typically, urban nursing homes operate with a skeleton crew on Saturdays and Sundays. In a facility downtown, for example, it is not unusual to find only one nurse on duty, whereas during the week there are four. Likewise, five aides will be on hand, as opposed to the usual twenty. The receptionist has also probably failed to show. By contrast, Forest Glen was always fully staffed on weekends. The laidback atmosphere of the rural facility belied the fact that competition was fierce, and jobs too scarce to jeopardize by calling off sick.

Aging itself was viewed and treated differently in the country than in the city. State regulations remained the same, yet geographic isolation did alter the way in which day-to-day obligations were met. It took a major hurricane to hit before the nursing homes that I served in the city would experience anything close to the tranquil atmosphere that pervaded Forest Glen on a regular basis. Urban power lines had to come down to reduce the volume of telephone and facsimile communications to the typically low level found in Forest Glen. As I made my rounds in the storm-hit city, the afternoon was peculiarly silent. The rain continued to fall, and the wind was high. I got a few faxes, and was paged once or twice but only regarding urgent issues. For once, I fielded not a single petty concern—nary a report on an unprescribed cough drop or a fall without injury. Insignificant matters came to a halt. The big storm in the city had forced us to focus on big problems, just as we did most days out in the country.

Staff in a Small World

Turnover at Forest Glen was low as well. When Lucy Barber retired as administrator, she had been on the job for several decades, and the change was momentous enough to stir into action the small corporation that owned the facility. After Lucy's big retirement party, the owners sent in Todd Carmello to see what was going on and to fix things up. Todd had grown up in the nursing care business. His parents had run a mom-and-pop rest home, and he was able to take what he had learned from them and combine it with the principles of modern, corporate long-term care. Come what may, he never forgot to see the business of facility management through the eyes of his parents, who had focused on quality care first and foremost.

Under Todd's administration all went well, as far as the staff at Forest Glen were concerned. The corporate brass, however, soon became displeased. Todd was supposed to be an unofficial spy and report on the ways that the facility was thought to be wasting money. Only he actually liked what he saw in the way of established care, and that was what mattered—was it not?—certainly more than the few minor discrepancies that he spotted in the books. If the staff at Forest Glen did not constitute a normal care team, Todd recognized that the level of care was excellent nonetheless.

Impressively, Todd succeeded in making his case at Forest Glen. He championed the facility and yet offered concessions to mollify the corporate owners. He cut costs but not at the expense of good care. With a unique blend of compassion and corporate know-how, Todd not only kept his job, he earned the respect of both his superiors and his employees.

As a whole, Forest Glen care team members complemented each other's idiosyncrasies and, like many a family, they managed to tolerate each other's shortcomings and sometimes even to enjoy them. Of course, there were exceptions. Some ongoing tensions were bound to originate far back in the shared history of a place so small and isolated, something I discovered as I learned more about the staff.

Not everyone was as sedentary as I had first imagined. True, Erin Caulfield was born and raised in Forest Glen. In fact, growing up, she had worked in the kitchen of the nursing home and later as an aide there. Yet she was a free spirit, who did what she pleased, not necessarily what pleased everyone else. Small town life bored her. She left home as soon as she could after high school. In the intervening years, she married and divorced twice, and mothered four children. She also graduated from nursing school and found a niche in long-term care in inner city nursing homes, mostly ones with a young and poor population. Time passed, Erin's parents grew older, and her life became more complex as she raised four sons alone, two of whom were biracial. In retrospect, some of her gripes against Forest Glen softened; other irritants she could no longer remember. Decades later, she returned to her home town. She came back to become director of nursing of the local long-term care facility at about the same time that Todd Carmello came on board as its administrator. If Forest Glen was a small village, the same might be said of a big city's neighborhoods. In fact it was in one of them that Erin and Todd first met and worked together for many years. The good vibrations of their harmony created a positive ambience once they met up again in Forest Glen in a welcome bit of serendipity.

Louella Green, on the other hand, had never lived outside Forest Glen. A licensed practical nurse, she had worked at the facility for nearly thirty years in one capacity or another. In fact, Louella was a high school acquaintance of Erin's. Unlike Erin, Louella was not particularly good looking. Pale and overweight, she tended to dress down in ill-fitting clothes and run-over shoes. Like Ingrid Cantor at Mission Hill, Louella did a good enough job not to be scolded but not good enough to receive recognition. Small town life suited her. Had she been presented with the many options of city life, I suspect that she would have become eccentric. As it was, there was something troubling about Louella, although no one could say why exactly. Pleasant and innocuous though she appeared to be, she had a few quirks. No matter what job Louella did, she finished it quicker than anyone else. She rarely asked for help, even if there was a problem, and she managed to find a solution on her own, although not necessarily the best one.

The physicians of Forest Glen were a unique bunch and a mixed breed. On the one hand were the locals, who had been there since the craft of medicine had begun, and they passed on the practice to their sons and, on rare occasion, to a daughter. The rest were outsiders, who had come to Forest Glen to express their dissatisfaction with the drawbacks of city life, or else because they had trouble fitting in socially anywhere. Bill Tomokhok was one of the latter kind of doctors. He did not care much for other people, and not too many cared for him either. He had been an engineer before he went to medical school, and it was unclear why he had decided to change career paths and enter a caring profession. Some people said that he made the switch after some trauma in his life, but no one knew what had happened. Ironically, Bill was not a bad physician and, among those that disliked the paternalism of country-style medical practice, he offered a refreshing alternative. His outpatient practice thrived, even if folks in Forest Glen had placed very low odds on his success when he first came to town.

Bill's attitude did pose problems in the nursing home, however. He did not like regulations. Not one merely to disregard the rules, he flouted them and acted out in fits of childish rebellion. He would, for example, write four-letter words on pharmacy recommendations, which formed an official part of individual medical records. He also came to see patients as he pleased and when they needed him but never in accordance with the monthly requirements set out by the state. In the city, most facilities would have asked him to leave, given his flagrant disregard for regulations. In Forest Glen, however, physicians were far fewer. A doctor would have to commit a major crime to be forced out of practice. We, Bill's colleagues, had little choice but to work with him. Discussion usually did not resolve much, but Dr. Bill and I had many conversations.

In another small-world coincidence, Bill had gone to the same medical school and residency program as I had, albeit a few years after me. In fact, I vaguely remembered his name, and then a colleague reminded me that we had been the preceptors for a resident clinic program in which Bill had participated. The distinction between city and country, which had once seemed so sharp, blurred a little more.

Like Bill Tomokhok, Laura Flamm was another city transplant to Forest Glen. She was a retired police officer, who at the age of fifty earned a degree in recreational therapy and went on to work in several of the city nursing homes, where she and I had crossed paths on occasion. Eventually, she arrived out at Forest Glen and became its activities director. When I asked what prompted her to relocate, she said that city life was stifling. I did not know what to make of that.

Laura was a hit with staff and residents alike. She came to work in costumes—bright pants, crazy tops, even pajamas—and had a knack for novelty that was refreshing in a town where even nursing home residents had little else to do but root for the high school football team. The team only played from September to December, however, which left a lot of blanks in the nursing home's recreation schedule. Laura filled them with activities that were interesting and joyful, and the atmosphere crackled with energy. What was normally unacceptable at Forest Glen became desirable if Laura was behind it. She spoke with the authority of a former police officer, even if she wore pink and purple polka dot pants and Cat in the Hat headgear.

Her people skills led her to also become the facility's unofficial mediator and, regardless of her lack of academic training, she was a capable mental health healer. Where she had come by her capacity to listen to people and help them resolve their conflicts was never clear, but no one particularly cared. Laura got good results, and we all saw her as irreplaceable.

Vendetta

Something had happened between Erin and Louella sixteen years ago. No one seemed to know the details, but everyone could sense the tension between the two. Shortly after Erin's appointment as director of nursing, Louella's mother, Sara Knightly, became a resident in the facility. For whatever reason, Louella chose Bill Tomokhok to be her mother's physician. No one approved of her choice.

Odd things began to happen with regard to Sara and her care. Items went missing from her room. On a number of occasions, staff discovered that her oxygen tank was set incorrectly, so that she either received too much or too little. Her medication list often got lost, or else a page might be missing so that Sara received erratic doses. How could so many mishaps befall the same person when the care at Forest Glen was relatively good? In the facility's thirty-year history, the number of errors associated with one person's care had never been so high.

Meanwhile, an odd thing occurred. Erin Caulfield's staffing records disappeared from her office. She never locked up, but why should she? She was out in Forest Glen, after all, where no one locked doors. Why take staffing records, of all things? They showed who worked on what day—nothing more.

When state inspectors arrived for a routine survey, Sara Knightly's chart attracted their attention, to no one's surprise. Each adverse event received painstaking scrutiny. The inspectors asked question after question, until they drilled down to ones that were quite specific: Which nurse worked the dayshift August 20 when Mrs. Knightly's oxygen tank was running full blast? Which aide worked the night of September 19 when the tank was barely functioning? Who was the supervisor during the day of September 20 when her medications were administered in adverse doses? Who was in charge of housekeeping and laundry the week of September 22 when Mrs. Knightly's nightgown was lost?

Now, of course, we saw how the two events converged—the negligent care of Sara Knightly and the removal of staffing records—the latter would provide answers to the inspectors' questions about the former. As to who did it, no one yet knew. Most staff members suspected Louella as the villain—she must have stolen the records to cover up inept care of her own mother. Erin Caulfield, meanwhile, was the victim of an embarrassing lapse, her basic competence called into question. Potential liability also loomed, given her inability to protect a patient. Most everyone at Forest Glen rallied around her, whose reputation they saw as unfairly placed in jeopardy.

A few staff members were unsympathetic. To them Erin was a prima donna that treated locals like second-class citizens. They viewed her as an outsider, tending to forget that she had grown up in town. Only a very few team members said nothing and kept their opinions to themselves.

As for Erin, she was not going to be taken down by events, not if she could help it. In fact, she would reproduce the missing staffing records. She enlisted the help of Laura, who as Forest Glen's activities director and unofficial team builder, came up with a plan. Every staff member that brought in time sheets for the two months in question would receive a paid day off. In addition, their names would be entered into a drawing for a $150 gift certificate at the local mall. Many people responded to the offers, and Erin was able to recreate a fairly accurate schedule, based on the information that they provided.

Erin also made a list of all those that had not turned in their time sheets. Louella was at the top, but not everyone else on the list aroused suspicion. Some staff simply had not kept their time sheets. A few could not be bothered. And a few, of course, had something to hide. Melissa Blackwell was a name that popped up, unexpectedly but tellingly. Currently the head of housekeeping, she had also held several other jobs, including one as an administrative assistant in the business office.

Another townie, Melissa was one of Louella's few friends, despite some ups and downs in their relationship. The two women were similar in many ways. Both were overweight and blowsy in appearance. Both had married several times to local fellows, and each had several children. In fact Louella's first husband was Melissa's second. In between husbands, and no doubt subject to a whole lot of other difficulties, Louella and Melissa had just recently decided to pool their meager resources and share rent on an apartment. Given the bad blood between Erin and Louella, it followed that Melissa and Erin were no friends either.

On the job, Erin had been skillful enough to supervise Louella and Melissa without reference to their shared past. Faced with a state inquiry, however, Erin made every effort to ferret out a motive for what had happened. That effort included revisiting old memories of her teenaged years, which were a blur, and for good reason. Erin had been a renegade then, and, unlike the calm and kind personality into which she had matured, the hormones of adolescence had lent her a mean streak. Erin and her boyfriend at the time had scrawled graffiti on Louella and Melissa's car (They were sharing things in high school also) and pulled a few other malicious pranks on the two girls. Although Erin had done nothing criminal, her behavior did inflict deep emotional scars on the two women, something that she knew but had never acknowledged.

Now, with the inspectors pressing her for answers, Erin faced her past and approached her two foes. She apologized for her long-ago misbehavior and asked Louella and Melissa to forgive her. To her relief, they did. For an instant all three women were sixteen again. Erin's sincere overture led to reminiscences, and a shared sense of reconciliation already had begun. The experience led Louella and Melissa to own up to their own wrongdoing. Louella had asked Melissa to remove the time sheets from Erin's office. For a friend as close as Louella, that was what Melissa did.

When the inspectors had arrived and found evidence not only of negligence but also of a cover-up, Erin was in a tight spot. Louella and Melissa admitted that they enjoyed seeing her squirm. Not only had she humiliated them in high school, she was top dog in their world now. Where was the justice?

Erin listened patiently. She thought that she understood how longstanding resentments could still simmer. What about all the things that had gone wrong with Sara Knightly, though? Did they have a hand in that too?

A silence fell over their interview as Louella nodded yes. Furthermore, what had gone wrong was not carelessness, she admitted. It had been deliberate.

Erin was horrified. Why would Louella put at risk her own mother's welfare?

The answer lay in an old secret. This hidden knowledge actually was well known, at least among the most die-hard residents of Forest Glen. Louella, it seemed, was abused as a child, both by her mother, Sara, and also by her father, by then deceased. Perhaps this sad experience explained Louella's oddness? In any case, she broke down and confessed. The opportunity to take revenge—first against her mother and then against Erin—two of her old tormentors—was just too great a temptation to resist.

The state inspectors were informed of the situation. Given the circumstances, they took a compassionate view. Sara Knightly had experienced no actual harm, Erin had reproduced the time sheets, and the culprits had confessed. The inspectors permitted Forest Glen to take responsibility for oversight and disciplinary action. Once again, the women were at the mercy of their old nemesis. Fortunately, Erin took pity on them to the extent that she could. She placed both women on probation. When Melissa said that she was too unhappy to stay, Erin helped her find a new occupation. In a town like Forest Glen, ways could be found to take care of one's own. Erin helped Melissa get a start in real estate. Interestingly, Louella chose to stay on at Forest Glen, even if it meant months of close monitoring and surveillance by the rest of the care team. In time, she earned the trust and respect of the other nurses. Her competence extended especially to the care that she took of her mother, Sara, in her last days.

Cold Ride to Death

I first met Iona Parker when she arrived straight from the local hospital. A little more than seventy years old, she was one of the town's retired school teachers, and had just been diagnosed with metastatic lung cancer. Because she lived alone and had no one to care for her, she came to live at the nursing home.

Iona was fairly pleasant and did not offer many complaints. She appeared resigned to her situation, which was a difficult one, involving both the chronic shortness of breath brought on by lung disease, and her cancer, which, of course, did not improve things. The staff, most of whom had known Mrs. Parker as a well-liked teacher during their school days, gave her special attention. They even wheeled her outside, as smoking was not allowed in the facility. Of course, these cigarettes breaks only worsened Iona's condition, and both Erin and Todd discouraged the staff from giving in to her cravings. Iona's prognosis was poor, however. Whether she smoked or not made no difference. When asked for my thoughts on the matter, I chose not to express a strong opinion.

Shortly after Iona's arrival, I received a call from her brother, Peter Blatt, a former research scientist, who had retired in Alaska. Rumor had it that he wanted to get as far away as he could from Forest Glen and still reside within the United States. Our conversation went something as follows.

"Iona went to Thanksgiving dinner with a friend of mine, who is a psychiatrist," Peter said. "He diagnosed her with depression. I don't want to impose, and you are her physician, but what do you think? Shouldn't you start her on an antidepressant?"

"Dr. Blatt, I'd be more than happy to talk to Iona about an antidepressant, but you know it takes a while for these medications to work. I don't think that Iona has that much time left."

"Yes, I see. Still, I'd like you to start her on one anyway. Let's make her last days happy ones."

"I'm willing," I said and then offered a suggestion of my own. "Visits from family might also lift Iona's spirits a bit."

Dr. Blatt chuckled. "I'm too far away to just drop by, I'm afraid."

"Yes, of course, but perhaps her son?" I was aware that Iona's son, an attorney, lived about an hour's drive from Forest Glen, about the same distance from the facility as I did.

"I couldn't say," Dr. Blatt said and rang off.

Staff members, who had grown up with Iona's son, had no explanation either—nothing that would explain his absence. It was left to a few devoted staff members to act as Iona's surrogate family. Fortunately, they offered her tender care and concern.

Iona began to decline very rapidly about three months after she had arrived at the facility. Peter Blatt called to enter his sister into hospice, with the written permission of her son, the phantom Paul. I recall the day exactly, because Iona's admission into hospice care coincided with a severe and dangerous storm. The city was paralyzed. As soon as the weather let up, the hospice nurse arrived to evaluate her condition and found that Iona had entered the dying process. Continuous care began. Someone from hospice was with her at all times, and I made sure that I was available by telephone at a moment's notice to ensure that Iona was kept comfortable with medications for anxiety and pain.

Forty-eight hours later, on the button, I received a call from Dr. Blatt. I returned his call immediately but was routed to voice mail. I was a bit annoyed. Why would he call me urgently and then not be available to take the return call? I left him a message to call me back. About thirty minutes later, he did.

"Dr. Silber, Iona's son would like to speak with you."

"Good," I said. "Please have him call me."

Dr. Blatt mumbled something about Paul not having my phone number.

"Well, please give it to him," I said and hung up to take a call from the hospice nurse.

"Iona is not doing well," she reported. "Her condition is becoming graver by the minute, but she is comfortable."

An hour or so later, Dr. Blatt called me again. "Dr. Silber, I've spoken to Paul. He needs to know what's wrong with his mother. Can you get out to the facility tonight? If you can't—and I know on a Friday night a long drive might be an imposition—Paul wants her sent to the emergency room for an evaluation."

I heard an ultimatum. Would reasoning work? My patience was at its limit. Still, I managed to keep my outer composure. "Dr. Blatt, Iona is dying of lung cancer. We've both known it for some time. There's no diagnosis to make, and a trip to the emergency room is not only inappropriate, I doubt that Iona would survive it."

"Paul is a very busy man," Dr. Blatt cut in. "He needs precise information. He needs to know exactly when to expect his mother's death so that he can schedule his visit. If you can't provide him that information, he's intent on sending her to the nearest hospital tonight."

"You must realize his request is ludicrous," I cried. "No one can pinpoint the hour of his mother's death. To send someone out in an ambulance in Iona's condition would be nothing short of cruel."

I made my point, but Dr. Blatt overruled me and called Todd Carmello. Whatever he said convinced Todd to call an ambulance. Staff members stowed poor Iona into the vehicle as a gale blew in and, with it, a heavy downpour. En route to the emergency room, she died as the storm's high winds buffeted vehicles on the highway.

I would soon learn that her son, Paul, had no regrets about the decision.

"His mother died on a mission," Peter Blatt told me. "That was how Paul saw it, and I think he was right."

In their eyes, Iona traveled to that emergency room for a legitimate purpose. She was going to get a real, science-based determination as to her condition—or die trying.

Life and Death Experience

Iona's death depressed me. So did those exasperating phone calls from her brother, not to mention her son's attitude, which had led my patient to die in a manner and place that I would have liked to have spared her. Exhaustion after a long week no doubt also contributed to the kind of dream state that I entered Friday evening when I was officially off the clock and could "relax." As I tried to absorb Iona's death, my mind took a strange turn. It does that, now and again, traveling mysterious pathways and making unexpected connections, to help me resolve things that are bothering me. This time my thoughts floated back to my children's births.

At the time of Iona's death, a local hospital was in the midst of a big advertising campaign to market its obstetric services. On my way to and from Forest Glen, I would pass a billboard that said "Have your baby at our home—Trinity." I found the sign vaguely disquieting, and soon I understood at least one reason why. A pregnant colleague had approached to ask me about my natal experiences. "Who was your obstetrician? What hospital did you go to?" She wanted to know.

When I explained that I had delivered at home with the help of a midwife, she replied, "Oh, I didn't know that midwives went to Trinity."

I tried to explain. After careful research and, driven by a strong intuition that the decision was right for us, my husband and I chose to have the births of all three of our children take place at home. I certainly have no regrets. The babies and I received excellent care from the assisting midwives, and I revel in the memories of how our family came to be. To my dismay, however, my colleague continued to conflate a home birth with one that took place at Trinity Hospital's so-called "home."

In the same vein, did Iona's son find it impossible to imagine death outside a hospital? To Paul's mind, apparently, death—like birth—was a medical emergency. For him, perhaps, last rites meant some form of procedure or investigation, even when to take action was a pointless exercise. To do nothing but watch and wait at a loved one's bedside was not an option.

At about the time that I first started to work out at Forest Glen, my eldest child began to study for her Bat Mitzvah. For a few months, most idle moments were given over to planning for this coming-of-age occasion, or else for the activities that would surround it. In fact, the drive out to Forest Glen actually came in handy, providing me with some quiet time to go over all the details and to anticipate catastrophes, natural or otherwise.

Of course I received plenty of advice from family and friends, but none of it yielded to the simple fact that this momentous occasion was our challenge. We had to successfully pass through the maze ourselves. True, we could have hired a professional event planner, but hiring consultants was not our style. Even if it were, we would still have been left with the worry. In addition to the mile-high list of things that I found to fret about, Abe managed to pile on a few more items. For weeks our imaginations were plagued by fears of what might ruin our daughter's rite of passage into young adulthood.

What if there was a tornado—would we be able to get to the synagogue? What if she made a terrible mistake and was embarrassed? What if her hair and makeup were not up to her expectations (She was a thirteen-year-old girl, after all)? How would the party go? Would the relatives get along? Would our careful seating plan reduce the chance of bickering or, God forbid, full-blown confrontation?

When the big day arrived, none of our fears came to pass. The morning dawned near to perfection—a balmy seventy degrees and sunshine in January—the weather not something that we could have controlled in any event. Shira's lecture was enticing in content and flawless in delivery. All of her friends were on hand, and the fun-filled party would make for happy memories. The only unforeseen event occurred when, unbeknownst to me, a few girls had gone into the temple bathroom to change from fancy dress to casual clothing, and I unknowingly walked in on four nearly naked teens. After all that planning and pondering, I was chagrined to be the central character in the only incident that involved screams of embarrassment. Still, the moment caused hardly a ripple in an event that went so smoothly. When it came to anxiety, Shira's Bat Mitzvah turned out to be the ultimate anticlimax. At the end of the day, Abe and I breathed happy sighs of relief. Weeks afterward, I still basked in the afterglow of our family triumph.

A few years later, our son stood poised for a similar rite of passage. He would have his Bar Mitzvah. Although the event involved about the same amount of planning and raised similar concerns, our fears were far fewer and less intensely felt than the ones that had surrounded Shira's Bat Mitzvah. Our son's day was just as perfect as our daughter's had been, yet the joyous aftermath was also a tad slighter the second time around. Like the first time on an amusement park thrill ride, Shira's Bat Mitzvah had combined fear of the unknown, adventure, and heady success at an emotional pitch that could not be repeated. Although we got on the ride again, we had the benefit of the first outcome to soothe us. If we still felt excitement, our memories helped to spark it.

My children's B'nei Mitzvah processes reminded me of how we, their parents, had long ago prepared for their debuts into this world. Planning, dreaming, hoping—and receiving plenty of advice and assistance—had all made successful births at home possible. What we learn from each other can be invaluable. Yet it has become clear to me that our experience is most authentic when the help we receive is woven into our own perceptions of reality. Experience is ours alone. If it were not, the world's many problems would not repeat themselves.

So how did Iona figure into these thoughts regarding the pangs of planning for major turning points in our lives? I think that the unfortunate way in which she died was the result of her son's desire to avoid direct emotional experience. Such a desire is widespread, of course, especially to deflect pain. By nature, of course, Iona had to do her own dying. Nobody could do it for her. Likewise, Paul lost his mother. There was no way to get around the fact, regardless of his success at shielding himself from the anguish of sitting by her deathbed in hospice. Although I mourned Iona's passing, eventually I came to mourn her son's avoidance of life as well. To avoid suffering and, perhaps any feeling, he had arranged to live in a comatose state. It was his mother who was dead, but he was half-way there himself. Poor Paul. For all the misery of my angst, I would not snuff out my ability to feel.

Birth and death mark the young and the old as vulnerable, hovering as they do near either end of the life cycle. They are most in need of assistance. How we treat them speaks volumes as to our own grip on reality. Do we face the inevitable, or do we try and duck and elude it? When it comes to life and death, will our children be able to learn just as much from what we embrace as from what we shirk?

Fooling with Fear

Major events in the life cycle, such as the death of a loved one, are known to put each of us at risk, physically and mentally. These radical upheavals in our lives translate directly into intense feelings, good and bad. No wonder that we tend to shield ourselves. Intensely real experiences can be hard to bear. One way to hide is behind synthetic emotions brought on by artificial perils like thrill rides, NASCAR, and television reality shows. My colleagues and I do something similar on the job, preoccupied as we are with care plans and management systems.

If "pretend" stressors appear to be on the rise, probably it is because they offer us the adventure of a crucial experience with relatively little risk. We may even escalate our sense of peril by taking on some actual form of danger, such as the kind involved in pursuing an extreme sport, going on an adventure trip, or participating in a reality show. None of these activities, however, carries the real weight of the risk, say, of going to war, undergoing major surgery, or perhaps even commuting on the freeway every day, for that matter.

As we seek to bypass—or at least numb—real trauma, however, the scary possibility is that we may begin to mistake our surrogate stressors for real ones. Recently, I came across an article about household remodeling. Much to my amusement—and dismay—I learned that home improvement is no longer simply a dream come true but now experienced by many people as one of life's major traumas—right up there with the anguish of death, the pangs of birth, or the high anxiety of job loss. Has luxury gone wild—or is it our fear of life's real ills that has?

Hoping to assure myself that the article just happened to feature a few unhappy people with singularly bad contractors, I read a little further on the topic. Alas, home remodeling as a social problem cropped up elsewhere as a trend, at least among America's upper middle class. Severe emotional distress could and did arise out of redecoration. Cautionary tales unfolded about couples reportedly divorcing over issues that arose during home improvement. If we were not careful, we could end up in a courtroom too. If, on the other hand, we managed to complete a home remodeling project with our marriage intact, we could mark the passage of another milestone in our pilgrim's progress toward self-improvement. As a precaution, then, should we perhaps seek a therapist to help us choose the right architect and the best building contractor? Designer drugs, meanwhile, have taken on a whole new meaning.

Next Stop Nirvana

Nursing home nomad Betsy Warner, as you may recall, was a past master at using pretend stressors to deflect real emotional stress and genuine physical deterioration. In fact, her various pretexts and pretenses were responsible for five out of the six moves she made to different nursing homes within a three-year period. Her move from Mountain Grove to Forest Glen was yet another stop in the search for "nirvana," or the perfect care team. Once more, I took care of Betsy, and we became reacquainted.

She was pleased to see me again, she told me, and relieved to find that nothing "terrible" had happened to me after Mountain Grove had asked for my resignation.

"I always knew you were a good doctor," she said. "I never really believed any of those horrid stories about you."

Fortunately, Betsy spared me the details. Instead she threw herself into life at Forest Glen. Having arrived around Thanksgiving, she quickly became active in the facility's festive activities as the holiday season got under way. In good health and high spirits, she became friendly with a few key staff members, including Erin Caulfield and also Laura Flamm, whose theatrical flare as activities director was much in keeping with Betsy's own. More surprisingly, Betsy developed a rapport with Louella Green. Louella had come a long way since her successful probation period, but she was still an enigmatic woman. Betsy also continued to rely on her daughters, who managed to visit her quite frequently. At base, it was family, not staff, who remained the bedrock of her well-being.

At Christmas, Betsy returned the kindnesses that she had received at Forest Glen by giving generous gifts to many members of the staff. She also paid for extra supplies so that Laura Flamm could expand on the whimsy and creativity of her activities program. Of course a few people remained in the cold, outside the blanket of Betsy's generosity, because they had not treated her quite as she wished. All in all, however, the holidays passed much to her satisfaction.

In the new year, Louella Green took sick leave to undergo surgery. Betsy missed Louella, whom she considered her personal servant as much as anything. The replacement nurse was perfectly competent, but an agricultural upbringing had not prepared her to deal with an urban sophisticate. The weather was poor, and Mrs. Warner's daughters did not visit much, although they phoned often.

Predictably, Betsy's moods declined. She stayed in her room and cried. The staff took her emotions in stride and paid them little mind. These farm-bred folks made sure that Betsy was comfortable, but they tended to recede when she raised a ruckus, confident that nature would take its course one way or another. This laidback attitude was a large part of the care team's passivity, something I had noticed when I first visited Forest Glen. Now I could see the wisdom in sometimes doing very little.

Eventually, Louella returned to the facility. Betsy was overjoyed to see her, and to tell her all that had happened in her absence, namely, the usual ups and downs, which by now had become all too familiar to me and Betsy's family. The aches and pains that Mrs. Warner had experienced during her absence preyed on Louella's mind, however. On her return to Forest Glen, she had come out of her shell to advocate on behalf of the woman that the rest of the staff called the "queen bee." Louella demanded to know why Erin had not kept her informed of Mrs. Warner's condition. She and Betsy had a special relationship, after all. And why, she thundered, had I not sent Betsy to the hospital for tests, as I had so many times in the past?

Of course I suggested to Louella that she sit down and read Betsy's thick medical history. Surely she would see the patterns and the pointlessness of further testing. Louella dismissed my idea. She placed no trust in medical records, which she knew could be massaged to say whatever the facility wanted them to say. Forest Glen was the least likely place for such a thing to happen, but Louella had heard stories about what could be done. She called the corporate hot line and complained about the facility. Her accusations, based on nothing, came to nothing.

Given Louella's past, Todd and Erin counseled the rest of the staff to show patience and compassion. No one objected, at least not openly. It was easy enough—and sad—to see Louella reach out to Betsy as a mother figure. Louella's was a classic case of the passive care team member, whose professional conduct undergoes a dramatic shift from general indifference to single-minded obsession with a patient or two. Still, most everyone remained uncomfortable with Louella's new intensity, at odds with Forest Glen' low-key environment. Privately, a few claimed that Erin still wanted to atone for bullying Louella in high school decades ago. Now the rest of us were forced to atone, too, they groused.

A Supporting Role

Louella continued to serve as Betsy's bedside confidante, and the rest of the staff continued to offer competent if impassive care—Forest Glen' trademark. Did Louella's presence really make a difference? Did her hand-holding and hand-wringing extend Betsy's life a little while longer? Possibly it did. If nothing else, Louella offered Betsy the kind of comfort that she preferred and appreciated. Yet in my experience, the care team plays no more than a supporting role in the individual's struggle with illness and death. The struggle itself remains a personal matter—and a personal responsibility—no matter whether the care team is utterly passive or hyperactive.

Our roles as caring professionals are limited for other reasons also. We operate with a Catch-22. We may genuinely care about our patients, yet we are bound by the regulatory and business requirements that apply to the institutional long-term care facilities that employ us. It was not my place to tell Betsy that she had so many somatic problems because she wanted to live with her family, not in a nursing home. Instead I was obliged to order diagnostic tests over and over again, with negative results to prove the point. Only near the very end of her life was I able to convince Betsy and her family to forgo the futile search for the magic cure. Our relative powerlessness as a care team was clearly evident in the case of Iona. We were unable to protect her from death in a cold ambulance once her son insisted on a trip to the hospital.

Having learned just how little I resemble a "free bird" in my profession, I long ago gave up my daughter Shira's fight to speak my mind without a second thought. Holding my tongue, I am left to wonder if we caring professionals have placed our "trust" in the long-term care management system to such a degree that we discount the value of our real-life experience. I wonder, too, if we not only dismiss but actually condemn our experience as a hindrance to good patient care. All I know for certain is that biting one's tongue is indeed a hidden hazard of my job.

Another Exit

Just because our influence as caring professionals is small does not mean that it is unreal. Betsy Warner did respond well to the steady care at Forest Glen, and to Louella's watchful presence. Yet the slow pace of life out there also led her to grow restless. When one of her daughters brought in a brochure for a fancy new facility in town, Betsy leapt at the chance to move back to "civilization." The "bovines," as she called Forest Glen's nurses, barely raised an eyebrow, as calm as ever in the serene setting, which Betsy chose to depart.

Thirteen
An Eye to the Future

Crescent Pavilion is a relatively new kind of residential care facility—patterned after a first-class hotel. Many that come here do resemble guests in terms of the length of their stay. (They undergo short-term rehabilitation and then return home.) Others settle into what is billed as a luxurious form of independent living. The relative few that need long-term care are housed in a private wing, hidden away from everyone else. For a time, Betsy Warner was one of them. She clamored to come live here, and basked with pride once she did. No wonder. Crescent Pavilion's grandness was meant for her, even if she was not well enough to enjoy most of its amenities.

Every inch a star, the Pavilion is spread across the top three floors of an architecturally handsome, five-story high rise. Upscale shops and boutiques occupy the lower floors. The arrangement is quite convenient, I suppose. If you tire of visiting your relative, you can always go shopping. Residents are encouraged to shop too. When they first arrive at the facility, they are greeted with discount coupons and a gift box of items from the building's retailers.

The street-level arcade includes a "Wellness Center," which does not offer medical or nursing services but rather the amenities of a day spa. There are also abundant opportunities to eat—whether fast food or haute cuisine—and to drink—whether at a coffee shop or a bar. In the lobby of the nursing home itself, a delicatessen serves grilled food and thick pastrami sandwiches. It is probably fortunate that physicians are on hand to prescribe an anticholesterol medication, if need be.

The dining room for short-term residents is exquisite. Soft-lit wall sconces and fresh flowers at every table create a sense of dining at a tony restaurant, often to the sound of live music. Guests order dishes off a menu, à la carte, and in the evenings they may enjoy cocktails at the open bar, set up in one of the lovely common areas.

Residential rooms are fully equipped electronically—Internet access, digital cable, cell phones, and plasma TVs. Still, the beds are small, and the quality of the linens, towels, pillows, and toiletries is institutional grade. Such a lapse leads me to wonder why anyone ambulatory, lucid, and affluent enough to enjoy life's luxuries would opt to choose independent living at Crescent Pavilion. The most obvious reason might be the specter of a sudden illness or incapacity. In other words, the independent come to live at Crescent Pavilion with an eye to the future. Enamored of the elegant décor and fine dining, they assume that they will be in good hands when the time comes for long-term care. Nursing, they assume, will be just as excellent as the wine that flows at dinner. Unfortunately, they overlook two facts—nursing care at the Pavilion is overpriced, and it is subpar.

The Cost of Beauty

Nursing care is overpriced and subpar largely because of the economic trade-off between the cost of beauty and the cost of staff. The price tag is bound to be high on a facility as well-appointed and amenity-filled as the Pavilion is. To maintain a profit, something has to give. In this case, it is the staff, just as it often is elsewhere. Doubtless, after a few complaints, the aforementioned narrow residential beds will be upgraded to something more capacious, and replacement linens will have a higher thread count. To absorb the costs, a few caregivers will probably lose their jobs.

I recall my last conversation with Angie, a young unit manager, who once handled medical appointments at Crescent Pavilion. "It's been nice knowing you, Dr. Silber," she told me, as I passed by the nurses' station on a Friday afternoon. "Today's my last day."

"I'm sorry to see you go," I said. "What's taking you away from us?"

"The new wallpaper that the facility is getting," she joked. "They need my salary to pay for it."

In her naiveté, Angie thought that she was kidding. In fact, she was quite right.

Designer wallpaper installation is one reason for the lean staff at Crescent Pavilion. Another is the emphasis placed on high technology and high security. Constantly upgraded computers continuously update residential medical records. All falls and other mishaps are relayed with electronic immediacy to the corporate lawyers. Surveillance cameras are posted at all exits and in the communal areas. Each exit also has a code that must be punched before a person can enter or leave the building. Residents themselves are outfitted with alarms, if they are deemed to pose a risk to themselves or others.

The latest gadget in use at Crescent Pavilion is a pager tree. It works as follows: A client (resident or patient) calls an aide. The call button is linked to a paging system. If an aide does not answer after two pages, five minutes apart, the floor nurse is notified, then the nursing supervisor, then the assistant director of nursing, then the director of nursing, then the administrator, and finally the owner's secretary.

The rub? Often no one answers at all. The various pagers wink and vibrate unceasingly while I do my own documentation by hand at one of the Pavilion's beautiful antique desks. As a last resort, I think, why not page the client's family? What would happen then?

On the facility floor where long-term residents are segregated, often I will find one lone nurse on duty to care for at least twenty-five people. All appears well—until someone becomes ill. In point of fact, however, all is not well. Short-handedness reduces staff contact with individual residents, which can be dangerous.

Not long ago I agreed to examine a man named Ted Bryant. When I arrived at the Pavilion, Mr. Bryant was not in his room. I asked a nurse to introduce us, as I had not yet met him personally. She had no idea who he was. The physical therapist did not know him either. Just before I had him paged, an aide came along, who apparently had helped Mr. Bryant that morning.

"There he is," she told me, and pointed out a man on the far side of one of the Pavilion's vast common areas.

As soon as I went over to greet my prospective patient, it became clear that the man did not answer to the name Ted Bryant. He was, in fact, Joseph Chapman, under the care of another doctor. Mr.

Bryant, as we learned later, had been away from the facility all morning. I was flummoxed, to say the least.

False Security

The security systems in place at Crescent Pavilion are first rate.
The trouble lies in the interaction between human beings and the
machines meant to do their work for them. As sophisticated and
sensitive as the facility's security system is, false alarms are a regular
occurrence. In turn, these initial alarms set off of a long chain of additional alerts and pagers. The constant bells and whistles have led to
complacency.

One evening, an alarm went off; then a second, third, and
fourth. The fact that no one responded was not unusual. What was
out of the ordinary, however, was that the alarms signaled a real emergency. Hours later, a staff member came upon a demented resident,
asphyxiated in the parking lot. Apparently, the poor man had lost
control of his runaway wheelchair, which dragged him up and down
the sloping lot in the rain and wind. Somehow one of the wheelchair's
safety straps had become wrapped around his throat and strangled
him. Both he and his conveyance were wired to set off alarms, if they
strayed any distance from the facility. Alas, technology alone could
only do so much.

Crescent Pavilion's lawyers succeeded in settling out of court,
and there were no real repercussions, not for the facility at least. The
Pavilion's owner had better connections in high places than the dead
man had with the staff. The "accident" received little outside notice,
and the facility continues to tout its cutting-edge technology for its
superior safety and security features.

Full House

Does the Crescent Pavilion manage to keep its beds full?
With ease.
Is there a waiting list for entry?
Often—and why not?
Official outcomes are good, despite the dearth of staff.
Outcomes are good because most residents are not really ill.
Many are "young" sixty-five year olds, who come to recuperate after
an elective knee or hip replacement. In fact, with some outpatient

therapy, many could probably go straight home—or else book a room at a fine hotel or take a leisurely cruise as they convalesced.

Recuperating post-ops are drawn here instead largely because of Crescent Pavilion's aggressive advertising campaign among physicians and discharge planners in hospitals. All Medicare recipients are entitled to skilled days of therapy in a nursing facility after surgery. Why not take advantage of this opportunity and come to Crescent Pavilion? True, a nice hotel, with meals eaten out, would cost ten times less a night. A cruise would be cheaper, too, as a way to rest after elective surgery. The scenery would be far more breathtaking, probably, and patients would be more likely to receive their medication in proper dosages, as they would administer it themselves. Problem is, such alternatives would have to be paid out-of-pocket. Neither Medicare nor Medicaid would cover such frivolity.

Keeping Up Appearances

As is typical in the industry, Crescent Pavilion is part of a conglomerate of nursing homes within a hundred-mile radius. Although each home is part of the corporate chain, variations among them are carefully cultivated to attract several different socioeconomic backgrounds. In the Pavilion's case, it is the most affluent that are wooed, and in particular those with minor medical problems and good insurance. The Pavilion relies a great deal on appearance, architecture, and décor to attract clientele. To some extent at least, it must rely also on the people it hires—people that will live up or down to the mission, image, and reputation that the owner wishes to promote.

The Pavilion shines as brilliantly as a diamond, and it is as hard as one, too. The polished surface of the unyielding stone reflects perfectly the personality of the man who owns the franchise rights to the Pavilion, Harold Muncaster. People who work for Harold must either share these traits, or else learn how to cope with them. Not surprisingly, the type of care team that has emerged at the Pavilion is a threatening one.

Typically, the ***threatening care team*** bullies residents and their families into accepting staff decisions and facility policy whether they like them or not. The team may issue warnings, such as eviction from the nursing home, should residents and their families resist. At the Pavilion, however, the threatening nature of the care team has turned in on itself as well. Certain staff members have taken it upon themselves to ensure that all of us comply with corporate decisions and policies even when we disagree.

Fred Lincoln, the Pavilion's administrator, does exactly what he is told. He receives his marching orders from Harold, reports to corporate staff, and takes no initiative as he manages the facility. Most of us on staff are keenly aware of Fred's impotence and do not want to embarrass him by asking him to risk doing anything out of line with corporate thinking.

Although he is a mouse behind the scenes, Fred is a standup comedian in the Pavilion's public rooms. Throughout the day he moves from one elegant salon to another to jest and trade quips with residents. Fred makes everyone chuckle. His congenial nature is a Pavilion asset—people enjoy him. Meanwhile, he has found that humor helps him cope with his lack of authority.

The Pavilion has a knack for hiring people that shine. If anything, Robert Lind was a bit too flamboyant for Harold's tastes. Still, he overlooked the fact, because Robert in his role as admissions coordinator managed to keep all of the rooms filled most of the time with desirable residents—ones in minimal need of care and possessed with excellent insurance. He also managed to keep a few names on the waiting list, should someone leave the facility earlier than expected.

Kind, reliable, and charismatic, Robert had no idea how poor the nursing care was at the Pavilion. How could he? Policy was clear: Robert was to book rooms, period. He was not to involve himself in the facility's day-to-day affairs. Once, however, he did answer a ringing phone at the empty nurses' station—and then followed through. Persistent and conscientious, he made a number of calls until someone could be found to help a resident in need of medical attention. Fred, however, was not at all happy that Robert had ventured beyond the confines of his job description, and warned him not to do anything like that again. Shortly thereafter, Robert resigned. He would have no trouble finding a position elsewhere. When Crescent Pavilion rehired, Fred was careful to choose someone like himself, someone who would not ripple the smooth surface.

Corporate Rules

Harold Muncaster prizes a smooth surface. He has a point. It would be difficult to maintain an image as glacially glamorous as Crescent Pavilion's without one. Yet Harold pleases himself, too. He hired an old high school buddy, David Dusseldorf, to serve as the medical director at Crescent Pavilion, and fixed things so that David also serves as the medical director of all medical directors within the conglomerate.

The main thing wrong with "Dr. D," as he is known, is that no one aside from Harold likes him—neither staff nor residents. Admittedly, he is a competent physician, yet he is also rude, overbearing, and vain. He yells at the staff and threatens residents if they dare to question any aspect of his diagnosis. In short, he is obnoxious. As Harold's friend, of course, he has job security without having to worry about pleasing the "clients." Someone else has to worry instead.

About six months after the Pavilion opened, the corporate administrators began to ask if I would take on more long-term care residents. Up until then I saw very few patients at the Pavilion, which runs a little rich for my blood and that of most of the people I tend to see. Corporate pushed, however. On the quiet, I was told that the facility stood to lose several long-term residents if I did not agree to see them. They had threatened to leave the facility if they had to remain under Dr. D's care. I was willing to oblige, and admittedly happy to be appreciated by my new patients. Yet I also felt used. There were strings attached, too. When I took on the very people that had rejected Dr. D, I was expected to abide by the care plans devised for them while under his care. A few times corporate suits chastised me for not using the facility's official forms to document my visits with patients. Worse still, they took me to task for not using the approved vocabulary on the approved forms. Corporate risk managers had carefully compiled an official list of terms from which I had deviated. How did they know?

When it comes to enforcement, the corporate office has an unlikely "ally," namely, Noreen Fabe, laundry supervisor. Noreen takes an avid interest in patient medical charts and regularly retires to her cubbyhole with a batch, which she is known to read as avidly as a summer beach novel. When I asked Fred why a head laundress had access to medical charts, he seemed unsure himself, although he told me that it had something to do with inventory. Eventually, I confronted Noreen, who was only too pleased to warn me that she likes to chat with corporate staff—"off the record, of course"—about medical staff failures to use the *right* vocabulary. From that point on, I understood that Noreen was sure to read all the notes that I made in my patients' charts. Although she hopes to catch me out, I take special care not to give her the satisfaction.

The constant surveillance has left me feeling bitchy, however, especially once I saw just how desperate the Pavilion's nursing situation really is. As I took on Dr. D's patients, I came into more frequent contact with Adele Sandler, the Pavilion's highly competent director of nursing. Adele had once worked at Serenity Acres, where our paths crossed briefly. She had not stayed there long. A facility as dysfunctional as the Acres did not especially prize competence, and had refused to give her more than a few hours' leave to mourn her father's sudden death. Adele went on to have a successful career elsewhere. Recently, however, she had suffered a few personal setbacks. When she was ready to re-enter the workforce, she vowed to find a job to last until retirement.

Poor Adele. She, too, fell for the Pavilion's beauty and paid the price. Her nursing staff is tiny and incompetent. Corporate policy limits her budget severely, which makes it impossible to supplement her staff with skilled or at least fresh recruits. When some of the better nurses quit, their jobs went unfilled. Those who remain have grown sloppy from overwork. Before long, Adele and I experienced a sense of déjà vu—as though we had gone back in time together to work at Serenity Acres. Her nurses fax me x-ray results that are two months' old. They call me about patients not under my care, or no longer on the premises. Some nurses cannot even pronounce the medications that they ask me to verify.

Templates of Caring

The limitations on nursing are not only financial. Just as headquarters insists that I use preapproved vocabulary to write up medical charts, they dictate the form of care that Adele and her staff are to provide. No longer do they sit down to discuss and develop plans to suit each individual long-term resident. Instead they check off boxes on a preprinted form that corporate provides. The check-marked items constitute a plan; once again, there are to be no deviations.

In fact, the corporate risk managers are toying with the idea of copywriting their preprints as "The Templates of Caring." According to them, there is not a problem that cannot be addressed by using one of their templates—noncompliant patients, belligerent families, smoking, wounds, constipation, drug reduction, malnutrition, you-name-it.

Crescent Pavilion seems to solve every problem with a piece of paper. Life might actually be touted as risk free, given all the efforts to prevent the unforeseen. No one could be malnourished, as they are given a vitamin. Other medications are prescribed liberally to ward off lawsuits—not so much illness. Defensive medical practice is the reason for these treatments, not medical need.

Devotion Amid Cynicism

Given the straitjacket in which Adele is expected to operate, she does her best to make up for it. Together she and I made sure, for example, that Betsy Warner was kept comfortable, as Parkinson's disease began to make serious inroads into Mrs. Warner's physical condition. Given the dearth of staff, Adele also is fortunate to have on staff two excellent nursing supervisors. Ellen Faust is remarkable in her ability to sidestep Dr. D, the Templates of Caring, and related requirements, unless they can be used in ways that have real meaning in her day-to-day practice. Devoted to her patients, Ellen spends long hours in the facility, compensating for the skeletal staff, and dutifully performing both direct patient care and providing proper documentation. She would work around the clock if she had to. Very much a mother figure, she also looks after everyone on staff—housekeepers, aides, nurses, and doctors alike.

Married three times, Ellen's last husband was said to be some thirty years her senior. He died a few years ago. Rumor has it that Ellen used to be involved in drugs. Her two daughters are social misfits and have been arrested numerous times for trafficking in illicit substances. One of them made Ellen a grandmother at an early age.

Some question Ellen's "Florence Nightingale" behavior, but I think that her underlying motives are to cure her own loneliness and to build self-esteem. Over time I have come to value her as a colleague, ally, and good friend.

Jill Kotsovas, by contrast, is a "nuts and bolts" nursing supervisor. In her own brazen and brash way, she is as kind as Ellen, but she can be slapdash when it comes to hands-on care, and her disdain for documentation is overt. Her real strength lies in befriending residents and their families. She makes it her business to sit at the bedside of those few people that die at the Pavilion. As she does so, she might read a travel catalog (Disney World is her favorite spot) or balance her checkbook, but she is there to hold a hand. At one point, she considered becoming a hospice nurse, but the paperwork involved was worse than at the nursing home. Besides, she asked, how could she capitalize on someone's demise?

Like everyone, Jill is bound by the Templates of Caring. Rather than sidestep them the way that Ellen does, Jill confronts them head-on and with a certain carefree cynicism. When it comes time to establish a care plan for a patient, she quickly checks off a few boxes on one of the preprinted forms and hopes that it will fly. Usually, it does. Crescent Pavilion's corporate administrators are as cynical as she is.

Reliance on canned care plans is a reflection of Crescent Pavilion's investment in the superficial. Yet there is something more to the investment than that. As is already clear, the facility sets its marketing sights on relatively healthy individuals with good insurance, who are in need of short-term convalescence after elective or minor surgery. With regard to actual nursing care, the corporate game plan is to identify medical problems among residents that can be solved readily. A perusal of the care plans in place at the Pavilion not so long ago revealed, for example, that most long-term patients were undergoing treatment for depression and gastritis. The high success rate on outcomes after treatment is advertised constantly to boost the Pavilion's reputation and to market the facility. No wonder, then, that Crescent Pavilion has put so much time and money into carefully crafting and enforcing the use of its care plan templates.

An Ugly Incident

Earlier in this chapter, I mentioned an unsuccessful attempt to meet a prospective patient by the name of Ted Bryant. Eventually, Ted and I met but not until after much uproar, which I learned about later in great detail. A healthy, outgoing man of sixty-four, Ted entered the facility to convalesce after elective hip surgery—just the sort of client that the Pavilion's marketing representatives have in mind, at least on paper. Everyone assumed that Mr. Bryant's stay at Crescent Pavilion would be brief and unremarkable. It did not turn out that way. Complications set in, including infection, an adverse reaction to antibiotics, and antibiotic-induced infectious diarrhea. Ted was hospitalized several times and then sent to the Pavilion's long-term care wing, where he was put under the care of Dr. D.

Not surprisingly, Ted was anxious to return to his normal, active life. He had many questions about his condition, which Dr. D was unable to answer. The problems that stemmed from the surgery were unexpected and not easy to diagnose. For his part, Dr. D was unaccustomed to discussing serious medical uncertainties with a patient that had the wit and the nerve to ask him searching questions. His responses were curt and apparently not at all forthcoming. Ted complained to Adele Sandler—loudly. Dr. D was discourteous, disrespectful, and, in a word, obnoxious. Ted wanted another physician on the double.

When Harold's assistant called me, I had just left town for a ten-day vacation. I agreed to see Ted as soon as I returned. It was Adele's unenviable job in the interim to keep the patient from jumping ship or creating unpleasant scenes. Her biggest challenge, of course, was to mobilize a shoestring staff of uneven quality to carry out the task. Ted had a big personality. He was not willing to sit and wait quietly for events to unfold. Over the next few days, he grew more and more restive while the nurses grew less and less obliging. Ever protective of her "brood," Ellen Faust threatened to walk off the floor if something was not done about the situation. Adele put in another call to Harold. The next thing she knew, Dr. D ordered a psychiatric evaluation for Ted. When Ted's wife found out, she was furious. She said that Dr. D needed one himself.

As tensions rose, Dr. D and Ted got into a real shouting match. One of the younger nurses fled the scene in tears, while another came in to see what the matter was. She threatened to call security and have Mr. Bryant escorted out of the facility for disrupting the peace. If Ted had been able to walk, he would have left the Pavilion there and then.

It was Jill's bedside manner that was the saving grace. She sat down and went over Ted's medical records with him and his wife and sympathized with the set of unknowns that they faced, given the cascade of complications. She helped the couple set up several appointments with offsite specialists in the area. Best of all from Ted's standpoint, Jill heartily agreed that Dr. D's care plan was mostly beside the point.

When Dr. D learned that his order for a psychiatric evaluation had been ignored, he went ballistic. He terrorized the entire nursing staff and then took his complaints to Harold. Harold got Fred Lincoln on the phone and ordered him to arrange an emergency conference. The next morning Adele, Fred, and Ted Bryant's wife and daughter assembled in the Pavilion's impeccably appointed conference room. Although the meeting had been hastily arranged in response to his angry complaints, Dr. D declined to attend the meeting. All things considered, it was probably just as well.

While freshly brewed coffee and croissants were served, Fred started in by offering his condolences with regard to Ted's ongoing problems, including an infected knee joint, clostridium-difficile colitis, anemia, fatigue, and now depression. Then he told the family that he understood that, for the sake of convenience, Ted would like to stay on at the Pavilion while he consulted several nearby specialists.

Ted's wife nodded in agreement. The offices that they needed to visit were an easy drive from the Pavilion.

Fred then commenced with the hatchet job that he was hired to do. Dr. Dusseldorf had ordered Ted an anticholesterol medication, he began. It was prescribed as a precaution to avert any heart problems. Yet Ted flatly refused to take it. His refusal, Fred claimed, was just one example of the risks that he was posing to himself and others through his uncooperative behavior.

"Ted has a hip problem, not a heart problem," Ted's wife responded. "I don't see why he should be forced to take the medication if he doesn't want it. How does that put anyone else at risk?"

"There are a whole host of problems, Mrs. Bryant."

"Like what?"

"Your husband refuses to follow doctor's orders. He refuses to follow his care plan. He places unreasonable demands on the nursing staff for time and attention. He's emotionally abusive."

"Abusive?" Ted's daughter was skeptical.

"He's made the nurses cry, and he disrupts the lives of his fellow residents."

"Well, he's not happy either," Ted's wife said. "Maybe we should find another place for him to stay."

"No," his daughter disagreed. "It's too much trouble until we know what's going on." Then she turned to Fred. "You've got to get that doctor off his back. Dad's ready to sue him, for emotional distress, if nothing else."

"Oh, I wouldn't talk about suing," Fred told her. There was a group touring the facility the other day, and they passed by Ted's room. "Boy, did they get an earful."

So if Ted sued, the Pavilion was prepared to countersue for lost business opportunities on account of his outrageous behavior. "Mr. Bryant's behavior left everyone aghast."

Ted's daughter managed to laugh. "I wasn't serious about suing," she muttered. "I just want to make Dad comfortable when he's having such a helluva time."

Where was Fred's famous humor, I wondered later, when Adele filled me in on the meeting.

Apparently, he was too intent on saving the situation to find time to crack a joke. "We're willing to make allowances," he went on. "It's true that to move your father now would be inconvenient and possibly risky, given the fact that it's not yet clear how serious his complications are. He's welcome to stay, with one condition. He must abide by Pavilion policy."

"What policy is that?" Mrs. Bryant inquired.

The care plan, Fred answered. Ted would have to stop complaining and start taking the antidepressant and the anticholesterol medication prescribed for him by Dr. D.

The following morning Ted's wife and daughters managed to take Ted out of the facility in a wheelchair to see the first specialist. When Ted returned to the Pavilion that afternoon, he and I finally met. Within minutes, we could see that we were going to get along. Together we would brainstorm how to devise a more appropriate care plan. Within the week, one of the specialists was able to determine Ted's post-operative problem. Within the month, he went home with what we hoped was a slightly more nuanced impression of the Pavilion. With Dr. D out of the picture, the rest of us did everything we could to compensate for what had been an unusually hostile and threatening experience for a short-term resident at the Crescent Pavilion. Harold, of course, knew how to dispel any lingering rumors about what had happened and otherwise saw no need to change a single thing about nursing care at the Pavilion.

Magic Medicine

The Pavilion's approach to nursing home care is no aberration but a reflection of current trends and developments. As we have seen, the care that is given often is determined based on the solutions that exist. Perhaps if Ted had gone along with Dr. D's prescription to lower his cholesterol, he would have felt better, at least on paper, as predetermined by the Templates of Caring. Guidelines have become very liberal. No doubt Ted met enough criteria for Dr. D to make the diagnosis legitimately.

But Ted's refusal to take the medication is not typical. On the contrary, the desire for a magic pill—either to swallow or to profit from—drives our expanding use of anticholesterol medications. Originally intended to treat the relatively few that suffer from metabolic problems, these drugs now are touted as cure-alls for everything from obesity to heart disease to premature death. Every year changing guidelines allow us to lower the threshold for treatment, to the point that we now prescribe to a large portion of nursing home residents a drug meant to combat a rare form of illness.

So widespread is the belief that the anticholesterol medication is a new cure-all that I have seen elderly patients on their deathbeds barely able to swallow, while their family members stuff the statin medications in their mouths only to be regurgitated a bit later. If what I have witnessed sounds deranged, it is a scene that goes into reruns every few months in my practice.

I have had a grieving daughter come to me—not for comfort but for reassurance—that the death of her father at ninety-five had nothing to do with him missing his anticholesterol medication on the day that he expired.

"Was that the reason he passed, doctor? Should I have tried harder to have him swallow the pill?"

The fervor that surrounds this medication is almost religious, with some people apparently prepared now to worship at a "House of Lipids," a sort of temple to ward off abnormal blood chemistry. Yet there is more to coronary disease, cerebrovascular disease, and diabetes than just bad fats. Increased cholesterol is only a small portion of cardiac disease. Blood pressure, obesity, inactivity, and genetic factors are also pieces of the puzzle.

Ten years ago, the standard of care was to counsel patients regarding life style and risk factors. A monthly follow-up to check progress was the rule. Now things have changed. A blood test and a slightly elevated value are all that is needed to diagnose high cholesterol and to prescribe a pill to lower it. No need anymore to recommend that your patient make a change in life style, although life style is the root of the problem. In fact, to do so is tacitly discouraged, because such a recommendation is not marketable, profitable, and is labor intensive. The magic bullet is indeed the magic pill. Drug companies sell a specialized and expensive medication to a huge population. Physicians bill to treat a huge population with the diagnosis. Insurance companies charge higher fees in order to cover so many more patients.

There are a lot of winners, but there are losers, too. The magic pill is not without its adverse consequences. Reality is not trumped.

The reality is that a few individuals—those truly in need of the anticholesterol medication—are camouflaged within a large pool of diagnosed people, who either are not really diseased or who would benefit much more from another intervention.

The patient that is not diseased may suffer the side effects of anticholesterol medications.

The overweight patient, who would benefit from exercise, may instead rely on a false sense of security derived from the diagnosis and the medication.

And, of course, even if insurance pays for the pill, the expense is passed along to everyone.

A Demand for Distortion

The treatment of illness can be manipulated in many ways. The common cold, caused by a virus, is widely and mistakenly believed to be treatable by antibiotics. Antibiotics are for bacterial infections, not viruses. Although public health officials and doctors alike have attempted to educate the public as to this distinction, it is not un-usual for people to visit a number of physicians until one gives in and writes a prescription. Competition in the medical field is brutal, and medical professionals often are under pressure to provide "customer satisfaction," never mind what is scientifically or ethically correct.

The consequences? Many drug-resistant bacteria have emerged. We no longer have simple antibiotics to treat common bacterial infections. Once rare bacteria are becoming commonplace. We have created a real life-threatening diarrheal illness (clostridium-difficile) which can kill the ill and infirm. Ted Bryant experienced this illness as an unexpected side effect. So did my former patient Imogene Mac-Dowell, who contracted it as a consequence of her quest for a cure for old age, which she and her daughter went on to pursue with another doctor. Have we learned? Are we curbing our use of antibiotics? Hardly. If anything, our dependence is only growing. Antibacterial soaps, lotions, and wipes are the norm. Increasingly, clostridium-difficile afflicts healthy people in a milder form—in part because we have mismanaged treatment of nonlife-threatening viral respiratory illnesses by prescribing antibiotics.

A Diagnosis to Deceive

Depression, once never spoken of, is now very much in vogue. In many states, it is a common clinical indicator, and the expectation is that at least fifty percent of nursing home residents will be on an antidepressant. Interestingly, nursing home regulators have come to see depression among residents as a plus, because the more residents on antidepressants, the higher the rating a facility is likely to receive for responsive patient care. To confound matters, state regulators typically require nursing home physicians to downgrade the dosage of the antidepressant medication every six months, or else to document the reason why.

Are nursing home residents really so depressed? Aging and the problems associated with the end of life certainly correlate, and even a relatively young and healthy person like Ted Bryant could slide into depression after post-operative complications left him in a state of limbo for quite a while. The aforesaid pressure to prescribe the many designer drugs on the market also explains the widespread diagnosis and prescription of antidepressants. Perhaps a third reason that we turn to the diagnosis is to hide flaws in family function and in the long-term facility care team—that is—a deficit in real caring.

Antidepressants are not cure-alls either. They are certainly helpful, and perhaps lifesavers in some cases. They should not be used alone, however, but in combination with other simpler, but labor-intensive modalities such as psychotherapy. Finally, antidepressants often take six or more weeks to take effect. Prescribing them to dying patients, as I am often "expected" to do, is of no actual benefit, other than to serve the pretense of care. A deathbed prescription might soothe an anxious family, and satisfy the needs of care planners, state surveyors, and drug company representatives—but not the patient.

Our growing reliance on a quick pharmaceutical fix is an insidious social problem, with consequences found far beyond the confines of our long-term care facilities. As more of us enter old age and infirmity with fewer coping mechanisms built over a lifetime, we will have little choice but to rely on prescriptions, subject to flimsy care plans with unforeseen results. In choosing drugs, we might well be left without excitement, enthusiasm, and vitality in the time remaining to us. In popping pills, we might well be left with no real means to reconcile ourselves to life's truths—which include death.

Ill by Choice

Alongside such challenges lies another. A new category of illnesses has emerged, what I call "diseases of choice." These illnesses include ones that arise, for example, from the excessive use of tobacco, alcohol, drugs, and food. All involve at least some element of personal volition, even if complicated by other factors. Obesity is one of them. There is a simple cure—eat less and exercise more—yet few obese people carry out this self-cure, and doctors have little financial incentive to encourage them to try.

Out of this new category of disease has emerged a new category of medicine, namely, treatments for diseases of choice. Gastric bypass surgery and smoking cessation aids are among them. Will these procedures help in the long run? We really do not know yet. In addition to the unknown potential that such aids have as curatives, other questions arise as to the broader and more indirect implications of such an approach.

What does undergoing a gastric bypass say to our children? Will they grow up to assume that they need not necessarily take care of their personal health? In the back of their minds, after all, they know that there will always be a pill or a procedure to ease any adverse consequences of their own abuse of their bodies. Will our children depend even more than our society already does on technical interventions to cope and survive?

Obesity has made itself felt within the long-term care facility, as a partial cause of a great number of chronic illnesses—hypertension, coronary disease, and diabetes. Yet, all by itself, the condition has helped fill many nursing home beds, much to the benefit of nursing homes financially.

Weight loss is medically advisable when it might enable an elder with osteoarthritis to walk, or perhaps to help him avoid a hip or knee replacement. Yet weight loss triggers a red flag among state surveyors as a signal that facility care might be poor. Ironically, it is not uncommon for nursing homes to give an appetite stimulant to any morbidly obese resident fortunate enough to have lost a few pounds. Of course, it is the indicator—and not the patient—that is being treated.

Self Help v. Real Help

Whenever I visit a bookstore, I tend to look at the shelves devoted to my own field—health and aging. Invariably, I am distraught at titles that trumpet diets that reverse the aging process, life styles that reverse the life cycle, and surefire ways to live a century beyond our births. Obviously, these books cannot turn back the clock. Just as obviously, these books sell, and there seem to be an endless number of them, separated by a year or two between each publication date. Our human hope that somehow we can avoid aging and escape death appears just as endless too.

The crucial aspect of each book, I notice, is some sort of punchy motto that will hook readers quickly and ensure the publisher a profit, even if the book's premise is off base. When it comes to aging and dying, honesty may not be marketable.

The care plans that play so prominent a role in facilities like Crescent Pavilion bear a resemblance to these best-selling self-help paperbacks. An answer that has helped a few is marketed to many. Any dilemma can be solved in ten steps, just as care for an aging individual can be determined by checking a few boxes on a generic list.

For better and worse, illness and aging are complex processes. Does anyone move through these life stages with greater ease after reading one of these self-help books? Surely some readers do but not many. It is their publishers, or perhaps their authors, who benefit for the most part.

Once again, I wonder how our approach to aging and dying will influence those that come after us. Have we set off on a path that our children can use for themselves and then extend—or will they inherit from us a bridge ready to collapse? Do we give them real care as they grow, or do we fall back on assumptions rather like the Pavilion's Templates of Caring?

Even as I raise these questions, the Crescent Pavilion thrives. Its glittery surface is so appealing. Betsy Warner remained happy there, right up until her eldest daughter retired and decided to give home care a go again. Betsy left the Pavilion with mixed feelings. Just knowing that she resided in a facility with a high glamour quotient had given her a lift. Still, her last days were contented ones in her daughter's home, where, unlike at the Pavilion, she could drink champagne, nibble hors d'oeuvres, and devour chocolate—all without a care plan. Her daughters made this contentment possible, of course. Without a family willing to step up and take responsibility for her care, Betsy might have met an end far less pleasant. Certainly it would have been far more constrained.

Fourteen
What Doctors Do

Doctors are supposed to preserve and prolong life, of course; that is our reason for being. Advances in medicine and technology have raised expectations of us further still. Today, it seems, any physician worth his or her salt should be able to cure any illness whatsoever and keep death at bay indefinitely. If nothing else, doctors at least must appear to alter the course of illness and death even in cases where all we can do, really, is work at the margins. I wonder: Does catering to unrealistic expectations cause all of us—doctors, patients, and families—more harm than good?

I had time to think about such questions one Friday afternoon as I sat and waited for our staff meeting to begin in the conference room of the medical practice that I share with six other geriatricians. Every quarter, the entire GeriMed staff gathers to assess where we are and what needs doing. The agenda reads pretty much the same from one meeting to the next. What does strike me each time, however, is how little my fellow physicians and I have to say in how we practice medicine. These meetings are largely formalities in which we sit mostly in silence to listen to Sharon Suttles, who was introduced earlier in this book, and who handles our marketing and customer services, and to Peter Knight, director of senior services for the Fountain Alliance system, with which our practice partners.

Marketing our medical services is not something that we GeriMed physicians have any particular ethical misgivings about per se. What we do object to is promotional campaigns and sales tactics that take on a life of their own, without necessarily an accurate reflection of what is offered. Sometimes medical products and services are promoted aggressively even before they actually exist. With Sharon in charge, our own small practice has nothing to worry about in terms of integrity. She fully supports our mission to offer excellent services and simply has no need to stoop to dishonest or misleading sales tactics. Creative, and gifted with interpersonal skills, Sharon is more than willing to work in concert with us physicians, at least to the extent that various regulations and the policies of our corporate parent permit.

Peter Knight is another story. Like Sharon, he has a degree in social work. Later he earned an M.B.A. By osmosis, he also seems to think that he picked up a medical degree, surrounded by doctors as he is everyday. Yet he devalues what we do.

"The doctor's primary role," he once told Sharon, "is to funnel patients into our hospitals."

Career for a Chameleon

Peter and I first crossed paths about fifteen years ago at a small nursing home where he was the administrator, and I was the medical director. Although I talked to him by phone many times over the first six months of his tenure there, I had never met him in person. He spent most of his time "out in the field," and operated more like the facility's marketing representative than its administrator. He showed up daily at area drop-in centers for the homeless and visited the local hospitals, where he plied the discharge planners with small gifts, such as coffee mugs and tote bags. A dreamer, he envisioned billboards all over the city to entice the elderly and infirm. Unnaturally preoccupied with the possibility of radio and television advertisements, he sought a way to tap into these means of communication to create a long waiting list, which all by itself would enhance the little nursing home's reputation.

I finally met Peter in person after he put in a frantic call to me one evening. State was due in first thing Monday morning to inspect the facility's records, and he needed copies of some reports of mine, which I had supplied four months previously but had since gone missing. The documents were ones that I could easily retrieve from my laptop. When I offered to drop them by the facility on my way home, Peter was appreciative.

A short time later I rang the buzzer to enter the building. It was after six, and the administrative staff had gone home. One of the night nurses let me in. She could handle the receptionist's duties af-

ter hours, given the facility's modest number of patients. I knocked
on Peter's door. There was no answer. The lights were out, but the
door was slightly ajar. I pushed it open with the idea of leaving the
requested documents on his desk. As I did so, I caught sight of him in
the far corner, engaged in a compromising activity with an attractive
woman. I stepped back from the doorway, and dropped the reports at
the receptionist's station on my way out. What had happened embarrassed me, and I wondered why he had left his office door unlocked.
Here I had been feeling guilty about not personally introducing myself to Peter and welcoming him to the facility. Now I felt blessed to
have retained my anonymity.

I still have no idea if Peter caught sight of me that evening. My
hunch is that he did not—but would not care if he had. In any case,
I steer clear of recriminations and accusations whenever I can. You
never know who your next boss will be, I always say.

Peter, however, had no medical training. He could not possibly
become my boss—or could he? In any case, he did not last long at the
facility where we met. Rumor had it that he overspent the budget
on a chronic basis. Other rumors surfaced regarding his sexual dalli-
ances, specifically with the owner's wife. He was let go.

Over the following years, I was to remain aware of the twists
and turns in Peter's career, if at a distance. Undoubtedly, he has a
great talent for landing on his feet. Although he has never held a job
for long, he has always found a new and progressively better one to
jump into just as he was about to lose the one that he had. About five
years ago, he landed the position at Fountain Alliance that brought
us back into direct contact again.

Right away I could tell that Peter was a different man. No longer
sloppy and unreliable, as he had been when he phoned me for those
lost records at the eleventh hour, he was seen now as a consummate
manager, attuned to the details, and sufficiently fair-minded to be
well-liked and respected. His latest and quite substantial promotion
had even led him to put aside his lewd ways, at least for the time being. In other words, Peter had changed his spots. His chameleon-like
ability to adapt and survive was what had remained the same.

Rube Goldberg's QA

This particular Friday afternoon, however, Peter was running late on account of the length of an earlier meeting over at the hospital. Could we just sit tight for a few more minutes, the receptionist came in to ask. None of us would dream of trying to reschedule. It was hard enough to agree on a date for these quarterly meetings in the first place. Long ago we had learned to build in a cushion on our calendars.

As I sunk down deeper into one of the upholstered chairs, I thought back to our last GeriMed staff meeting. Then I had been poised to take my recertification exam in internal medicine. There was no mystery as to why the exam came to mind. As usual, our agenda this afternoon would include discussion of our latest performance indicators, that is, quality assurance, with regard to our medical practice. Quality assurance is something that I tend to associate with my recertification.

As part of the process, I had to complete a performance module, which was largely a teaching exercise, and one based on the honor system. I did everything "by the book" and spent months planning, collecting data, and implementing my study unit. A friend, who was undergoing the same recertification process, was not as thorough. In fact, she faked her data, she told me later, because she was too busy to do the research.

Who got the better grade?

My friend did, by a long shot.

I scanned our latest QA results, attached to this afternoon's agenda. We had not faired too badly this quarter. In fact, our statistics were better than ever, probably because enough residents were on antidepressants, which state surveyors tend to consider a sign of good care. The important question for me, however, was whether our care actually was any better in fact. I would like to think so, but we provided excellent care long before laws mandated us into quality assurance. My experience and day-to-day observations led me to believe that the level of our care had merely remained steady. Yet our QA indicators varied from one quarter to the next. How could this be? To get an answer raised more questions.

How were the data obtained? Were the indicators themselves inaccurate, or was the collection of them errant in some way? As part of the QA process, the medical skills of each physician in our practice are tabulated and quantified by a data entry clerk with no more education than the clerk from whom we must get insurance pre-authorizations for our prescriptions. We have had trouble keeping such clerks on the job. So sought-after are they in our area that another medical practice generally will succeed in wooing them away with a higher salary. Thus each quarter usually it is a new person that sifts through our performance records to decide how we are doing. Seriously, we ought to consider doing a quality assessment on our quality assessor.

What has arisen from the institutionalization of quality assurance unsettles me. Among the unintended consequences are the communication barriers that have arisen among doctors, nurses, and their patients, along with a surge in distrust. The complaint chain that has replaced direct communication between medical professionals and patients leads to confusion, which breeds suspicion, frustration, and hostility. A simple question about quality of care now has to travel through a Rube Goldberg machine that is over-engineered to perform a simple task in a complex way. The time lag before the arrival of an answer, which may be unsatisfactory, leads to a complaint, which generates another question, which leads to bewilderment and anger. Yet this ridiculously complicated system, which health care employees must tinker with constantly to keep running, has become far more secure and "important" than the jobs that it is designed to "evaluate." In the process, standards of medical care seem to be created without the involvement of a doctor or a nurse.

Who gains from the QA process? Not the patient, the physician, or the nurse in my experience. Instead the guidelines largely seem to benefit the paraprofessional, a manager like Peter Knight, to help him gain some control over matters about which he knows very little.

The Market for Speed

A lack of knowledge has never stood in Peter's way, however. In fact, his directorship within the Fountain Alliance system gave him the confidence to become ambitious. Peter decided to create a comprehensive geriatric assessment center to provide thorough medical evaluations of frail elders. Typically, such evaluations are very labor-intensive and rank low on the reimbursement scale for physicians. From a business standpoint, Peter's venture thus was risky, as it was not likely to be a moneymaker. Yet he received full corporate backing. Given his position, the new center presumably would funnel patients into the Fountain Alliance system, just as we doctors at GeriMed were meant to do, according to Peter.

As bait on his lure, Peter built into his plans everything he could think of to make a visit to the assessment center a pleasant experience. The waiting rooms were to be spacious, well lit, and filled with comfortable seating. Soothing landscapes would hang amid flat-screen TVs. Coffee and light fare would be on hand, and patients that happened to be at the center mid-day would have access to a sumptuous luncheon buffet. It was no coincidence that Peter was friendly with the owner of the Crescent Pavilion. When it came to amenities, clearly he had borrowed from that facility's playbook.

Leery, I gave Peter the benefit of the doubt nonetheless. If the medical exams were good, all the extras would be fine. I even contemplated the offer of my own services at the new center a few days a month. In exchange, I could view geriatrics from another perspective and make a difference, if in a somewhat unorthodox way. As Peter developed his plans further, however, it became clear that my interest in volunteering was misplaced.

One day he gathered us GeriMed physicians together and explained the situation. We should be at the heart of the new center, he began. Many of the assessments would involve complex medical analysis, and we were the top geriatricians in the city, after all.

We waited for the other shoe to drop and drop it did. The problem was that he and his hospital backers planned to market the center largely on how quickly they could get tests performed and the results back to patients—quicker than anyone else around. So, Peter went on, physicians were needed that knew the Fountain Alliance system "inside out" to get the job done "fast." He made no mention of accuracy, I noticed, only speed. To run the center, Peter selected several doctors on the hospital staff, none of whom were geriatricians or had even had much contact with the elderly.

Fountain Alliance's CEO was enthusiastic. He stood ready to refer his own parents to the center once it opened. I myself felt downbeat, given the real possibility of subpar assessments. Yet what could I do? Powerful players on the business side of medicine had joined forces and held sway. I had to pick my battles judiciously.

The Controlling Factor

One battle that I did wage involved the hire of certified nurse practitioners, something that GeriMed colleague Jeff Wang and I wanted to do. A CNP has enough advanced training to assess, diagnose, and treat patients and to prescribe controlled medications. A physician's role can then be that of a consultant on cases that are complex. Jeff and I were at the point in our practices where it made sense to delegate some of the less challenging tasks. Although we were motivated by our desire to save time for better care, it was widely known that the addition of a nurse practitioner to a medical practice would cut costs and increase billing. Unsurprisingly, GeriMed Corporate jumped on the bandwagon and offered to hire our practitioners for us. In return, Jeff and I were to provide a sufficient workload to support the new hires' salaries and benefits, something that would not be hard to do.

I gave careful thought as to how Dr. Wang and I would interact with our new staff members, and how best to forge a collaborative relationship between corporate and those of us in the field. I came up with some terms that I thought would benefit all concerned.

Although technically employed by the GeriMed Corporation, each of the nurse practitioners would also work for each patient and family, as well as for Jeff and me. Any potential for conflicts of interest needed to be addressed at the outset. Meanwhile, however, emphasis on cooperation among all entities ought to be a priority.

As I saw it, the role of the nurse practitioner would be to provide expert medical care with the support and under the supervision of a physician. The practitioner's purpose was to supplement the care of a nursing home resident in ways that a floor nurse could not. Ideally, the practitioner would have the skills to enhance nursing and medical care and to help the facility thrive as both a business and an asset to the community.

What I did not want to see was our new hires simply do things that I or another physician had the time and the ability to do but would rather shirk. Likewise, the same should hold true of work that the nursing staff could do itself. With respect to the GeriMed conglomerate, the new hires should be made with a long-term role in mind, not merely as a short-term means to attract more income.

In anticipation of the interview process, I proposed two questions to be put to applicants:

1. The facility develops a care plan (for your approval). You believe that the plan is contrary to a resident's needs and wishes. How do you proceed?

2. A family member asks to speak with you about "something bad" regarding the facility. What do you do?

Later I would learn that GeriMed's corporate editor rewrote my questions, to read as follows:

1. What skills do you have to assist the facility in developing care plans?

2. What approach would you use to act as a liaison between facility and family?

After a flurry of e-mails, the situation became crystal clear. I had been naïve to assume that GeriMed Corporate would permit us physicians to oversee our nurse practitioners and provide advice and guidance day-to-day. My carefully wrought terms and conditions were never taken seriously. Corporate glossed over and then cast them aside. Jeff Wang and I would have no role in the interview process, no say in defining the position descriptions, and certainly no say in selecting the actual hires. We would work closely with the new employees, but we would not assess how well they were performing. We would, in other words, shoulder responsibility but wield no authority. We were simply to be grateful for what GeriMed Corporate paid for, no questions asked.

What to do?

In the end we did what I had wanted to do in the first place. Jeff and I would each hire a nurse practitioner ourselves. We would keep our independence and oversee how the new hires functioned. Fortunately for us, Jeff and I had practiced together for many years, and we trusted each other as we would a family member. Our decision to pay our own way obviously would be more expensive in the short term, but in the long run we would hang on to autonomy and integrity in the practice of medicine.

Death by Process

Our receptionist appeared at the conference room door again. Peter was on his way, she told us. Then she handed me an envelope. Inside it was a death certificate for Nancy Loomis, who had passed away several days ago. Rather than rely on snail mail, the family had sent a courier, who now waited in the lobby for my signature. As I took hold of the certificate, I recalled Nancy's passing. Her death came as no surprise. At ninety-five, she had had no real medical problems other than old age itself. Over the past year, she simply had begun to fade away gracefully. She had spent the last several months of her life in hospice, which gave her family added support with her physical care.

Hospice was legally bound to inform me of any changes in Nancy's condition, even though I was no longer doing anything for her curatively. The first time that the hospice nurse called, she told me that Nancy was in the "early active" stage of dying. I had little idea as to what she might mean exactly. A few hours later, she called again. By then Nancy had entered the "active" active stage. Meanwhile, as far as the family was concerned, Nancy was simply dying. Everyone had gathered around her bedside, to be present and mourn her passing.

After the hospice nurse rang off the second time, I stopped to wonder. Did pinpointing death's approach in a series of stages make any difference? Perhaps, I thought, the process helped to distract us, and hide us from our ultimate powerlessness? Still, the nearsighted focus reminded me more of modern obstetrics, which discretely but arbitrarily categorizes phases in a natural process. Everything was properly documented, the nurse assured me when she called the third time. I did not care much about the care plan, but I was relieved to hear that Nancy was comfortable and that her family was with her when death finally came.

With the courier standing by, I took a look at the certificate. The state required that I provide a cause of death on the form. I could choose from a number of options. Old age was not one of them. In our state, you could only die from something on a preapproved list. I had no choice but to improvise. Quickly I jotted down heart disease, signed my name at the bottom, and handed the certificate back to the receptionist.

Nancy's heart had, after all, stopped, I reasoned, which led me to recall what had happened with my patient Nellie Barnes. In her case I had chosen cerebrovascular disease as the cause of death. The family was so upset that they threatened to "kill" me unless I issued a new death certificate. They wanted me to write, "Mother died peacefully." I sympathized but referred them to the county health department that made the rules about what I could write. They never did come after me with a shotgun, so I guess I managed to convince them.

Theory and Advocacy

Death is a funny business, all the more so among those near the end of life. A former patient of mine, Marion Johnson, told me that she used to run a funeral home. I was intrigued. I had known many people in my career that were funeral directors, but I had never really discussed the profession with them. What, I asked, had drawn her to such a line of work? Then I remembered: Marion had moderate dementia. Probably she would not understand my question—and yet she did.

"I was looking for a job, and there was a need in my area for this type of service," she said. "Black people die more often than white people," she went on to inform me. Then she gave me a long look. "Are you Jewish?"

"Why, yes," I responded.

"You're lucky then. I've only done a few Jewish funerals."

Few whites and practically no Jews had lived in the largely African American neighborhood where Marion had grown up and, much later in life, was crowned "Homecoming Queen." As a middle-aged woman, she won the title as a show of appreciation for her professional services in a community that viewed dying as "coming home." Now dementia had come along to distort experience and observation, which led her to conclude that blacks died more often than whites and Gentiles more often than Jews.

I went on to ask questions about her medical history, that is, until I looked into her eyes and saw that she really did not understand at all. Marion did not seem to mind. She continued to surprise, even to catch me off guard, from time to time.

"Doctor, the old know what it's like to be young, but the young don't know what it's like to be old," she told me one day. "The young know that they won't get old or sick. Aging and dying—that's no problem. It'll never happen, so why plan ahead?"

I winced. You ought to come to some of the planning meetings at Mission Hill, I thought. Recently, I had sat there for hours and hours as we discussed how to handle the possibility of a pandemic flu. As I sat and waited now for the GeriMed quarterly meeting to begin, I was reminded of how much time medical professionals spend in meetings like these, planning for things that probably will never happen. The emphasis on the theoretical future requires us professionals to overlook problems that exist, here and now, but go unattended because we do not have the time. News headlines decry the shortage of nurses, but please do not forget that they are required to leave their patients' bedsides to sit in conference rooms and discuss hypotheticals.

No wonder Marion had remarked to me, "Why, I can't even get my teeth brushed around here, but what can I do?"

Clearly, she sensed the shortage of hands-on care, even in her compromised state. Sadly, her sense of helplessness is only too common. Yet Marion impressed me greatly, because she seemed to really grasp the fact that by the time we decide to advocate to age and die with dignity in nursing homes, we are usually too feeble to try.

All of this would discourage me, were it not for occasional rays of reassurance that radiated from patients like Jacob Eliot. He contracted AIDS in the 1980s and, like Marion, spent his last years in a nursing home where he echoed her laments. Yet the videotape of his funeral, which included a clip from a personal interview just before he died, filled me with a sense of redemption. I had made a difference, he said, as he looked out from the television screen with his soulful eyes. I was just what I aspired to be—a good doctor.

The Power of Drugs

I steered my mind back to our quarterly meeting. Not only had Peter arrived, he presided. He mentioned the upcoming symposium, which GeriMed sponsored each year on health and aging. As usual, experienced geriatricians would be passed over as speakers in favor of "hired guns," whom the pharmaceutical industry paid to jet across the country and give talks at various events like ours. Although the speakers offered the disclaimer that the pharmaceutical companies did not endorse what they had to say, we all knew better. No matter what the program stated, Topic A would be the latest drug that they were pushing.

Peter instructed us on how to conduct ourselves. We should be sure and stop and introduce ourselves to each drug representative at the symposium. They were doing a great service, he explained, and we needed to thank them and encourage their efforts. Although disgusted by Peter's words, they did conjure up for me Harry Simon, the one drug representative that I actually liked.

For the price of a four-dollar latte, Harry always gave me the insider's scoop on his world, where financial kickbacks were the norm and fudged data the means to an end, namely, to boost a drug's sales quotient. If, like many physicians, I felt bullied by drug reps, there was a reason. Drug reps were in sales, as Harry reminded me. Whether the drug was good, bad, or indifferent, their job was to convince me that it was desirable, would not cause patients to die prematurely, and should warrant coverage by insurance providers. No wonder they were aggressive and provided little useful information.

Hospital systems like Fountain Alliance often enjoy rebates and other discounts associated with the use of a sole vendor and the bundling of certain pharmaceutical products. So it was not at all unusual for a hospital manager like Peter to urge doctors, like us at GeriMed, to mingle with pharmaceutical representatives at a symposium. The "great service" that he spoke of would really amount to a negotiated settlement between our hospital and some of the companies. The drug reps, with whom we were expected to make nice, would steer us to the preferred products. If we declined to use them, the hospital might decide to look for physicians that would.

As the afternoon drew to a close, I felt low, but could not figure out if it was because my thoughts had turned to patients like Nancy and Jacob, who had passed away, or because of the sad truth spoken by Marion about the helplessness of people that live and die in nursing homes. Maybe it was the shamelessness that Peter displayed? Maybe it was because I knew that we doctors often did choose expediency; we went along to get along.

All of the above, I suppose.

God Needs a Risk Manager

Our meeting adjourned well after five o'clock. As I headed out the door, Peter complemented me on my jewelry, but his overture did nothing to make me feel better. Fatigue, I decided, fed my discouragement regarding nursing home care and my profession. Yet the underlying concerns that worried me were real enough even when I was wide awake. What did the *Templates of Caring* mean to a person who had just lost their loved one? Did it matter if a care plan was in order when death arrived? No care plan or consultant could prevent the inevitable, namely, death and the great sense of pain and loss that followed, nor could our care plans prevent what was meant to be. No matter how much we tried, our documentation would never capture the essence of any one person's life.

Before I wrote this book, I wrote another—*Living and Dying in a Long-Term Care Facility: Notes from a Nursing Home Doctor.* The book offered composite portraits of many of the people that I had seen as patients in nursing homes for more than a decade. To try and capture my innermost feelings about my professional experience, I mentioned several seeds of thought that led me to write a book in the first place. They rise directly out of my experience still.

Within the nursing home context, God (in the form of Truth and Fate) must be managed (handled, controlled, or directed) to minimize risk (of loss, misfortune, injury, disease or death). Although this observation reflects my actual experience, the attempt obviously is absurd. Of course God (Truth) cannot really be managed, yet that simple fact does not keep people from trying in their fervency to protect against risk. Fear gets its due and then some. The manager's hedge against loss takes precedence over ethical medical care for the elderly and infirm. We fight or else evade the immutable (old age and death) yet recoil personally from the very people that need our care as they cope with the end of life.

At the Mercy of Image

This current book focuses less on individual patients and more on the facilities and types of teams that take care of residents. During the time that I wrote it, two of the facilities where I once saw patients have closed. Three more have changed their names to help attempt an image makeover. The two homes that closed both took on difficult residents, including those that suffered from such problems as multiple chronic conditions, wounds, or persistent mental illness. One of them was Meadowview. The other home was not mentioned in these writings.

As I described earlier, my grade suffered during a recertification process because my performance module featured something less than the perfect data that my friend had invented for hers. Likewise, a less than perfect inspection record penalized two honest nursing home facilities but not the ones that cooked their books. As we have seen, working in a nursing home requires all sorts of resourcefulness to cope with rather rigid regulations on the one hand and smoke-and-mirrors on the other. I may not be permitted to state the real cause of death on a certificate, whereas an under-qualified physician can give elders a subpar examination in an assessment center whose only real merits are its decor and buffet table.

It was no coincidence that the two facilities that closed were not as well appointed as many other facilities in town. A bogus care plan and fancy wallpaper would have been better bets than the genuinely good care that they gave to risky patients, even if their paperwork was sloppy.

Should Meadowview and the other facility have hired a consultant, then, to solve their problems? Not in this case. There would be little point for homes that were as honest and unvarnished as they were. Today's consultants need not be experts in the fields in which they offer advice or facilitate change. Peter Knight, as we know, has no medical education and very little background in geriatrics. Yet he has offered professional advice regularly on how doctors should do their jobs. He has hardly seen a resident, let alone cared for one. His advice comes from the board room, not the exam room or the shower room, not to mention the nursing home where our patients live.

No wonder most care teams are dysfunctional. The team leader has gone to business school, not to medical or nursing school. Of all the facilities mentioned in this book only one, Mission Hill, has a normal care team. Again, it is probably no coincidence that the facility's longest serving administrator was a nurse.

Peter's career arc shows, too, how far the business side of medicine can remove us from the human side. Later on, he would change his spots again and leave GeriMed to climb the corporate ladder. He would forget all that he had learned about running a small local nursing home and building a team of geriatric specialists to serve a major hospital. Instead he would focus on consolidating and hanging onto to his own emerging power. Eventually, he would reach the pinnacle of his career and become the CEO of a mediocre nursing home chain, which he would miss no opportunity to promote. His compensation, as well as his status, would be what mattered. He would have too much to lose personally to worry about the quality of what his chain of homes had to offer.

When we enter a long-term care facility, or help our elderly or infirm relatives to do so, we strive to find a place that will feel like home. For the nursing home staff, that should translate into an effort to create a normal, functional care team, whose members have the personal virtues and the professional expertise to supplement, and sometimes replace, the care that a healthy family life should offer. Yet we succeed all too rarely, despite all the requisite planning and regulated activity.

If we want to experience this last path in our lives in ways that are satisfying, we must change fundamentally our philosophy of health and aging. A highly paid consultant without a medical background, who manages care through plans drawn up to minimize risk, is not what we need to make life more meaningful. As health care consumers, we will have to refuse nursing home care that does not serve us and our actual circumstances. Until we do, we will see little change. And we should act now. As Marion Johnson understood, by the time most of us need to advocate on our behalf, usually it is too late. We are already at the system's mercy.

Family

I began the long drive home feeling guilty. I would arrive too late to cook. The kids, at least, were ecstatic to learn that dinner would be pizza, defrosted and warmed up in the microwave. The cell phone has changed our lives. I relayed the news about dinner and learned what was going on at home even as I drove there. As I reflected on all that was going on in my children's lives, I was reminded once more of my former patient, Sally Ballard, whose altered sense of time put Christmas in February. For me, summer started long before June. May was a killer as three kids finished the school year. The exuberance and excitement of their youth filled the house these days, as thoughts of freedom from schedules danced in their heads. Yet even as we anticipated the last day of classes, we planned for June and July. There were summer programs to look into and reservations to make. By the time that August rolled around, we would focus on the winter holidays even as we got ready to go back to school, with its supply lists and, of course, a new batch of forms. Perhaps Christmas does come twice a year. Shopping, which I used to love, has become a chore. All this planning adds to my grueling schedule, while the passage of another milestone in my numbered days as a contented mother of young children can feel bittersweet. Perhaps the nurse practitioner that I was going to hire would ease my workload and make the road easier to travel.

I took advantage of my drive time to call Maude Hulse about our birthday lunch. She and I have known each other a long time and have developed the habit of celebrating our birthdays together. A former floor nurse, Maude now runs a nonprofit for nursing home residents in need and offers the kind of personal care and attention that I wish were commonplace. The funds that she helps raise are put to good use. They are simple nonessentials, but they can significantly improve life—cosmetics and hair supplies, colognes and aftershave, and fresh flowers and houseplants. Maude is the sort who would see to it that Marion Johnson had a decent toothbrush and would help her use it, too.

Because Maude visited nursing homes throughout our area, she was always able to fill me in on what was new. At Mission Hill, one of my patients told her today that he was ready to go home and manage on his own again. I doubted it, but should I let him try? Otherwise, Hillary Berwald, her old mentor and my ideal social worker, just moved to Boston to be near a new boyfriend. Maude talked to her tonight, and she was doing well, with the prospect of another job as an administrator. We would miss her very much. There was good news: Ludmila Sidorova had finally bought a house. The bad news: She lost her job when Meadowview closed, which left her scrambling, of course. More good news: She had several job leads already.

Halfway home, I said goodbye to Maude. As I drove on, my care team "families" faded, except, of course, for Carol Sue, to whom I would dutifully report the day's events once I flopped down on a sofa. My real family was waiting. At least I could still tell the difference. Sometimes I worry that society-at-large soon no longer will. Professionals are expected to act like "families." Why not the reverse? Will the preferred cough medication disappear from the nightstand unless a family belongs to a particular health plan? Will an elder be required to call a central number if she falls at home? Once she is seen to be at greater risk, will her insurance premiums rise, just as they would if she had been in an auto accident?

I gave my parents a quick call. The family scrapbook that I started last December sat on my desk at home. At the center was a photo taken then, one of the few of my mom and me. Usually one of us takes the pictures. Summer would begin and come to an end. In an instant it would be December. Maybe then I would have time to start in on the book again.

At last I turned into our driveway. As I entered the house, Abe stood in the kitchen, ready to offer me a glass of wine. I had better take it slow, I thought, as I had consumed very little that day—one Starbucks vente latte, one Diet Coke, and three chocolate-chunk granola bars. By a quick calculation, I arrived at six hundred calories. As I pulled the pizza from the freezer, I listened happily as my family gathered round and caught me up on their latest news tidbits. Shira was at work on her quilt, having received advice from my mother on how to correct a mistake. Avishav was done with the butterfly puzzle. Fluffy, Hoppy, and Latte, her three stuffed bunnies, were fed and ready for bed. Jared won his basketball game. He got a B on his science test but was well prepared, which is all that we ask.

Despite so much joy in my life, at the end of the day I am pulled down by a weariness that leaves me weepy. But I have no time to cry. Perhaps I could hire Doris Clayborn, the crying lady at Mountain Grove, to do it for me? Or do I really need a consultant, a manager, or a marketing agency to see me through? Not at all. I will get a good night's sleep and make my usual rounds in the morning. I will smile, despite some of the things that I have written here.